Healthcare
Innovation
Shaping Future Models of Delivery

Series on Technology Management

Series Editor: Joe Tidd (*University of Sussex, UK*)　　　　　　ISSN 0219-9823

The Technology Management Series is dedicated to the advancement of academic research and management practice in the field of technology and innovation management. The series features titles which adopt an interdisciplinary, multifunctional approach to the management of technology and innovation, and includes work which seeks to integrate the management of technological, market and organisational innovation. All titles are based on original empirical research, and includes research monographs and multiauthor edited works. The focus throughout is on the management of technology and innovation at the level of the organisation or firm, rather than on the analysis of sectoral trends or national policy.

More information on this series can also be found at http://www.worldscientific.com/series/stm

(Continued at the end of the book)

SERIES ON TECHNOLOGY MANAGEMENT – VOL. 43

Healthcare Innovation

Shaping Future Models of Delivery

Editors

Mona Seyed Esfahani
Bournemouth University, UK

Matthew Halkes
Torbay and South Devon NHS Foundation Trust, UK

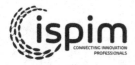

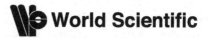

Published by

World Scientific Publishing Europe Ltd.

57 Shelton Street, Covent Garden, London WC2H 9HE

Head office: 5 Toh Tuck Link, Singapore 596224

USA office: 27 Warren Street, Suite 401-402, Hackensack, NJ 07601

Library of Congress Cataloging-in-Publication Data

Names: Seyed Esfahani, Mona, editor. | Halkes, Matthew, editor. |
    International Society for Professional Innovation Management, issuing body.
Title: Healthcare innovation : shaping future models of delivery / editors, Mona Seyed Esfahani,
    Bournemouth University, UK, Matthew Halkes, Torbay and South Devon NHS Foundation Trust, UK.
Other titles: Healthcare innovation (Esfahani) | Series on technology management ; v. 43.
Description: London ; Hackensack, NJ : World Scientific, [2024] |
    Series: Series on technology management ; vol. 43 | Includes bibliographical references and index.
Identifiers: LCCN 2023015007 | ISBN 9781800614185 (hardcover) |
    ISBN 9781800614192 (ebook for institutions) | ISBN 9781800614208 (ebook for individuals)
Subjects: MESH: Delivery of Health Care--trends | Biomedical Technology--trends |
    Diffusion of Innovation | Organizational Case Studies
Classification: LCC R858.A2 | NLM W 84.1 | DDC 362.10285--dc23/eng/20230607
LC record available at https://lccn.loc.gov/2023015007

British Library Cataloguing-in-Publication Data
A catalogue record for this book is available from the British Library.

For any available supplementary material, please visit
https://www.worldscientific.com/worldscibooks/10.1142/Q0418#t=suppl

Desk Editors: Logeshwaran Arumugam/Adam Binnie/Shi Ying Koe

Typeset by Stallion Press
Email: enquiries@stallionpress.com

Printed in Singapore

About the Editors

Mona Seyed Esfahani is a senior academic from Bournemouth University, renowned for her expertise in innovation adoption and communication. With a primary research focus on innovation in healthcare, she explores the dynamic intersection of healthcare and technology, studying ways to enhance the adoption and communication of innovative practices. As the Chair of the Health and Innovation Special Interest Group at the International Society for Professional Innovation Management (ISPIM) and Cluster Head for Communicating Health Innovations in Science at Bournemouth University's Data Communication Research Centre, Mona leads collaborative efforts with international partners to unravel the complexities surrounding innovation adoption, behaviour and communication within the healthcare industry. She is working on various projects with NHS partners, such as utilising Virtual Reality technology for pain management, developing interventions to improve patient journey and improving Health Innovation adoption.

Matthew Halkes provides clinical leadership for innovation at Torbay and South Devon NHS Foundation Trust, an integrated provider of health and social care serving the population of Torbay and South Devon, UK. His role supports the creation of organisational culture and adoption of innovation best practices that enable the Trust to achieve its strategic objective of continuously improving the delivery of care. A particular focus has been on the development and scaling of digital technologies that empower patients to self-manage their conditions (Health and

Care Video Library and the CONNECTPlus app) which has been achieved through the creation of a joint partnership venture, Health and Care Innovations. Dr Halkes acts as Clinical Director for the company, providing useful insights into the interaction between the public and private sectors. Within the Trust he has also been instrumental in supporting the creation of the Digital Futures. This incubator hub brings together clinical teams, academia and industry in order to explore the role of immersive technologies in healthcare. An important aspect of his role is connecting with regional, national and international networks in order to bring up-to-date knowledge of innovation methodologies and approaches into the organisation. This has included participating in the three-year EU-funded TACIT knowledge alliance project partnering with universities and companies (including Lego, BMW, Nokia, Generali and Lufthansa) from across Europe on the development of innovation training resources.

Contents

Introduction

In June 2019, during the International Society for Professional Innovation Management's (ISPIM) annual conference, the Special Interest Group on Health and Innovation was born. The aim of the SIG was to act as a knowledge hub for academics, professionals and businesses to share ideas and present research. The work presented in Florence was the starting point of this edited book series. Discussions around health ecosystems, managing innovative hackathons, health innovation solution development and management from academics and professionals around the world were extremely inspiring. So the journey started in early 2020, and as we all know, COVID started. Cucknell and Weir (2022), referred to COVID-19 as 'the greatest healthcare crisis in the post-war era, causing huge disruption to global medical systems'. As much as COVID has been a disruption, it has also resulted in a high demand for 'local and innovative solutions' (Barbosa *et al.*, Chapter 5). This book includes many traces of COVID, the impact it had on the health systems, the new innovative solutions that came to play in such a short period of time and how innovation management systems adapted to the new situation. As chapter contributors were identified during presentations in virtual ISPIM conferences, the book shaped and progressed. Yes, there were many pitfalls, COVID-related ones, which resulted in delays and dropouts, but finally, the book was completed.

This book explores innovation in the health sector, there are discussions on innovative technologies, covering development and manufacturing approaches and innovation management and training. There are case studies reviewing the successful application of innovation models and technologies from Brazil, Portugal, Austria, United Kingdom, Sweden and Europe. There is a close link between the healthcare industry's challenges during COVID-19 pandemic and how the industry has coped.

In the first chapter, Cucknell, Weir and Whittle (Chapter 1) share their perspective, as innovation consultants and practitioners in the commercial sector, on the impact of COVID on the health system in the UK and the lessons that can be drawn on for the future. From this unprecedented shock to the healthcare system new models of delivering care rapidly emerged enabled by the accelerated adoption and scaling of a range of existing technologies (such as telemedicine and drones) into practice. The authors reflect on the conditions that enabled this rapid adoption to occur, but also highlight some of the issues that unless addressed may affect the sustainability of these changes. They then describe a projection of what healthcare could look like in the future if this momentum was maintained and digital healthcare technologies, ranging from AI to robotics, were developed and implemented to their full potential. They reflect on the conditions required to enable this to happen, including the new business models and suggest that this will lead to a 'blurring' of traditional boundaries of who provides care.

Polónia and Gradim (Chapter 2) examine the question of whether an innovation management system can bring additional value to existing processes. Through a case study of two state-owned hospitals in Portugal (one medium-sized and one a larger institution), they assessed that although innovation is identified by organisations' senior leadership as a key strategic priority, there was little evidence of a systematic approach to innovation management. There is limited investment into the resources (human and financial) and infrastructure required to manage both internally generated innovation and external partnerships effectively. Monitoring and evaluating the impact of innovation was also identified as a neglected area.

They observe that the system struggles to move from a "'command-and-control' to a more orchestrated approach involving all stakeholders and participants (Pikkarainen, Hyrkäs and Martin, 2020; Polónia and Gradim, 2021). The consequence in these institutions is that innovation projects tend to be largely driven at a departmental level, often with external funding, with the attendant risk of misalignment with organisational priorities and dispersion of innovation efforts. The picture is not completely negative with evidence of some human capital policies to support and reward creativity, and one institution has a Research, Development and Innovation (RDI) unit responsible for developing and implementing innovation management processes. They identify that although the literature in healthcare is limited and a potential area for future research, effective innovation management can positively affect a hospital's overall performance. They outline a suggested road map for achieving this goal.

Kihlander, Nydahl and Vlachos (Chapter 3) review the 10-year journey (2011–2020) of increasing innovation maturity at Karolinska University Hospital in Stockholm, Sweden. One of the largest university hospitals in Europe, Karolinska has a worldwide reputation for excellence and is ranked 6th in *Newsweek*'s list of recommended hospitals (*Newsweek*, 2023). This journey is outlined in a number of phases from the creation of the Center for Innovation (CfI), proactively leveraging value from partnerships working and prioritising capability development through to developing a holistic systems approach to innovation. They reflect on the issues and challenges associated with adapting and implementing innovation management approaches into the public healthcare setting, where exploration of new opportunities can't interfere with the daily delivery of care. They highlight that centralised formal management approaches can run the risk of decreasing drive and creativity as well as the need to combine top-down and bottom-up approaches. They challenge the perception that hospitals are primarily adopters rather than generators of innovation (motivated by the challenges faced in everyday practice). While recognising that there is no one specific model that meets all requirements and therefore the need to take an open approach, Kihlander *et al.* recommend a number of areas that can be developed with respect to innovation in healthcare based on their experience. They emphasise the importance of taking a holistic systems approach that brings together strategy, process, performance and a culture of 'organisational innovativeness' (Salge and Vera, 2009) rather than simply focussing on implanting an innovation management system. There also needs to be a focus on knowledge sharing among hospitals, more focused funding and collaboration between practitioners, patients, academia and policymakers. A pertinent observation is that the innovation support function should never lose sight of the future.

Hackathons are often used in open innovation approaches to bring together internal and external participants in the development of potential solutions to identified challenges. However, they can be inconsistent in the results they generate. Sadr and Granig (Chapter 4) present lessons learned from a non-systematic literature review of hackathons from a range of sectors, including healthcare, and the factors that increase the likelihood of them being productive. They also present the advantages of embedding hackathons into the Vienna Innovation Model (VIENNO). This model, developed by the Vienna General Hospital, VAMED-KMB, and the Carinthia University of Applied Sciences, is a holistic approach that draws on the expertise available in an established innovation ecosystem in which there is shared awareness and knowledge of the system challenges and where collaborative working is fostered through investing in social capital. VIENNO offers a patient-centred, cross-functional result by hacking the old processes and delivers purposeful and future need-based innovations through co-sensing, co-inspiring and co-creation (Sadr and Granig, 2019). This innovation ecosystem approach provides a framework that enables the efficient organisation of hackathons that have increased reliability in terms of productive outputs. The combined effect is to enhance the capacity of system players to meet the current and future challenges facing healthcare through being able to respond at speed and have a clear vision of the future state.

The adoption of innovation in healthcare is often difficult and slow due to the complexity of the sector. Not only are there multiple stakeholders, users and benefactors but also parallel systems, roles and procedures. Barbosa *et al.* (Chapter 5) describe a unique case of vastly accelerated delivery of an innovation driven by the extreme and critical need generated by the COVID-19 pandemic. The result was the development of a regulatory-compliant medical device (a ventilator) from design to manufacture in an incredibly short time frame and at low cost. The authors have identified that this required the orchestration of rapid network mobilisation, within and across organisations, driven by the common mission created by this public health crisis. They have identified that a critical factor for success was individuals taking on 'assumed roles' that were not defined by their predefined job description, but by their knowledge, skills and personal networks. This organisational adaptation from a strategic-oriented approach to a rapidly responsive, economic and flexible approach (Chapter 5) enabled risks to be mitigated, resources acquired and the project to be delivered at pace. They observe that this experience provides transferable learning to nonturbulent conditions. Those organisations that actively invested in embedding themselves in knowledge-rich networks and who understand the augmented capabilities of their staff are likely to be much more able to respond rapidly and effectively to less acute but equally important challenges.

To meet the challenges of the pandemic, there was a need to rapidly and efficiently train and educate healthcare professionals to take on new 'assumed' roles. This needed to be delivered within the constraints associated with minimising the opportunities for virus transmission. Ghatnekar *et al.* (Chapter 6) talk about how the use of Technology-Enhanced Learning (TEL), and specifically Virtual Reality (VR) and Augmented Reality (AR), was successfully used in a UK NHS hospital (Torbay Hospital, Devon). TEL has been proved to facilitate knowledge acquisition and improve decision-making (Guze, 2015) and can be customised to deliver a personalised experience, which was a necessity during the COVID-19 pandemic. Learning technologists, clinicians and educators came together and used a pragmatic design thinking methodology in order to develop solutions that could be implemented within a time frame that met the immediate need. Use cases highlighted include supporting staff being redeployed to unfamiliar settings, the acquisition of new skills (such as doffing and donning of Personal Protective Equipment (PPE)) and maintenance of staff well-being. TEL has also played an instrumental role in maintaining undergraduate and postgraduate medical education during the pandemic through facilitating remote teaching and training (Goh and Sandars, 2020). Ghatnekar *et al.* (2022) discuss how these use cases could be transferred to other healthcare providers and the learning gained extrapolated to support workforce development in the 'new normal'.

Continuing the immersive technology theme, Heydari Khajepour *et al.* (Chapter 7) examine the use of VR as an innovative therapeutic intervention in pain management and specifically explore its effectiveness in the area of acute pain. Poorly managed acute pain not only has significant implications for the individual affected but also for the healthcare system as it is associated with increased risk of complications and progression to chronic pain, with the attendant higher use of healthcare resources. There is significant interest in the potential role of non-pharmacological interventions such as VR and AR, and this has evidence of being effective in some patient groups such as burns and dentistry (e.g. Sharar *et al.*, 2007; Felemban *et al.*, 2021). Heydari Khajepour *et al.*'s literature review highlighted that there is a good body of evidence for the impact of these technologies, but that the current studies have some limitations. Reassuringly no negative effects have been identified. They suggest that further research needs to focus on patient selection and the influence of particular elements of the experience, such as level of immersion and interactivity, on the impact seen. They also highlight that there is the potential for adoption of these technologies in multiple branches of medicine — not just pain management.

As outlined in Chapter 1, a variety of healthcare technologies will play an increasingly important role in future care delivery. ALMEDA (Tageo and ALAMEDA H2020 Project Consortium, Chapter 8) is a three-year Horizon 2020 Research and Innovation Framework Programme which brings together an international collaboration of clinicians, software developers and researchers with the intention of accelerating the deployment of digital healthcare technological interventions, specifically remote patient monitoring and next-generation AI, into practice. Their focus is on enhancing the delivery of value-based personalised healthcare in the neurological conditions of Parkinson's disease, multiple sclerosis and stroke. In Chapter 8, the authors outline the significant health burden presented by these brain conditions, the challenges they present to healthcare professionals and the potential benefits that the combination of multimodal patient monitoring coupled with Big Data analytics and AI algorithms can bring, in terms of the delivery of personalised assessment, treatment and rehabilitation resulting in improved outcomes and quality of life. The data provided to healthcare professionals by these technologies will support diagnosis, the monitoring of disease progression (including the ability to predict relapses and detect deterioration early) and provide the ability to assess the impact of the existing and newly developed therapeutic interventions, both positive and negative. Sharing of the data captured from patients between individuals and teams involved in their care will facilitate true integrated multi-disciplinary working. Healthcare systems will benefit from cost-saving service efficiencies through process innovation, improved insight into population health needs and the potential to address workforce shortages.

The chapter summarises the findings of the first year of the project, which has focussed on mapping the current care pathways at the three participating pilot sites with an emphasis on understanding current usage of digital healthcare technologies, the maturity of integrated care models and the extent to which shared decision-making is being used to support the delivery of value-based healthcare. An important aspect of this baseline information gathering has been the identification of the potential factors that could either enable or hinder future development and deployment of solutions in the different national contexts the project is operating in. The authors stress that pathways of care will only be truly transformed if these healthcare technologies are adopted into practice, which requires them to have a high degree of end-user acceptability and usability and then delivering clear value and benefit. Critical to achieving these objectives is the prioritisation of end-user engagement throughout the innovation lifecycle, selecting use cases that represent the population that will be using the tools developed in practice and co-designing solutions that directly address their needs. This human-centred design approach is regarded as particularly important in digital healthcare where the rapid pace of change brings an attendant risk of losing sight of the patient perspective and the opportunity to benefit from their experiential knowledge. The importance of end-user engagement has led to its inclusion in published codes of conduct and regulatory documents in the UK and Europe. Although the ALMEDA project focuses on three important neurological conditions, the challenges they present to patients, carers and healthcare professionals (as well as wider society) are representative of many non-communicable long-term chronic health conditions. The learning from this project, both in terms of accelerating the uptake of digital healthcare technologies through creating the conditions that support development, evaluation and adoption, as well as the specific tools developed, will have eminent transferability to other contexts.

The resilience and responsiveness of healthcare systems and their ability to reconfigure or transform services to meet acute and chronic challenges and meet the diverse individual needs of patients are often dependent on the availability of medical supplies. Usually operating in the background and largely unseen, it is only when the traditional supply chain fails, as seen during the pandemic with shortage of PPE and ventilators, that this dependency is brought into sharp focus. In Chapter 9, Kapletia and Phillips introduce Redistributed Manufacturing (RDM) as a transformation from a 'current state' to a 'future state' typically involving a shift away from large-scale centralised manufacture towards small-scale decentralised manufacture and geographically unconstrained supply chains, operating closer to end-users/beneficiaries to produce personalised products, on demand, with less waste and stockpiling (Srai *et al.*, 2016).

Although at an early stage of maturity in healthcare, RDM has the potential to play an instrumental role in transforming future models of healthcare service delivery (Mueller *et al.*, 2020) and delivering significant impact. However, its adoption requires system change across business, manufacturing and medicine. Kapletia and Phillips propose that the complexity of RDM and the routes to adoption are best understood through the lens of transdisciplinary innovation. This conceptual framework provides an integrated systems perspective. It is a powerful tool for providing insights into the factors that affect innovation development, adoption and performance, particularly in the context of complex or 'wicked' problems that have societal importance (exemplified by healthcare). The authors propose that applying the transdisciplinary innovation analytical approach can answer research questions on the healthcare system's preparedness for adopting RDM and identifying where it could have most impact. They identify that transdisciplinary innovation methodologies could have equal utility in other contexts within healthcare, such as the adoption of new technologies or the development of innovation capability.

Summary

Even prior to the COVID-19 pandemic, global healthcare services faced escalating demand driven by the combination of an ageing population, increased prevalence of long-term health conditions and increased expectations with respect to equity of access and outcome. This, combined with the constraints imposed by limited financial and workforce resources, was a significant driver to developing the innovative new healthcare delivery models that meet the quadruple aim of improving population health, enhancing patient and healthcare professional experience and achieving financial sustainability. COVID-19 continues to significantly impact health services through not only the need to treat patients, but also vaccinate the population. This is compounded by the backlog of care that has been created over the duration of the pandemic. The crisis during the acute phase of the pandemic saw significant innovation occurring at scale and pace. The need to continue reshaping the delivery of healthcare has not gone away.

We hope that the contents of this book will be of interest and value to academics, healthcare professionals, innovation practitioners and businesses as well as those involved in setting strategy and policy. The involvement of all these players will be required as we address the important societal challenge of equitable access to effective and safe healthcare. Individual readers will take away different learnings depending on their personal perspective shaped by the context in which they work and perhaps the maturity of their current innovation systems and processes. For the editors of this series, one of the consistent themes that has emerged is the importance of diverse knowledge-rich networks has being critical to supporting successful innovation. These networks need proactive curation and management in order to create value for each of the players and deliver an amplified wider benefit to the ecosystem they support. Their facilitation may require modification and adaption of current regulatory and governance frameworks. Another strong message is that those organisations that had a foundation of prior exploration, experimentation and early-stage implementation were better placed to deliver accelerated adoption at scale when required. This is aided by enabling staff to work to their strengths (skills, knowledge and creativity) and allowing them to be motivated by their interests rather than limiting them to a tightly defined job role. Business models and access to research and innovation funding also have an important role to play in both enabling the development and testing of new propositions and the widescale adoption and spread of those with proven value.

References

Cooper, N. (2021) World's Best Hospitals 2021. Retrieved from https://www.newsweek.com/best-hospitals-2021.

Felemban, O. M., Alshamrani, R. M., Aljeddawi, D. H., *et al.* (2021) Effect of virtual reality distraction on pain and anxiety during infiltration anesthesia in pediatric patients: A randomized clinical trial. *BMC Oral Health*, 21, 321.

Goh, P.-S. & Sandars, J. (2020) A vision of the use of technology in medical education after the COVID-19 pandemic. MedEdPublish (Preprint).

Guze, P. A. (2015) Using technology to meet the challenges of medical education. *Transactions of the American Clinical and Climatological Association*, 126, 260–270.

Mueller, T., Elkaseer, A., Charles, A., Fauth, J., Rabsch, D., Scholz, A., Marquardt, C., Nau, K. & Scholz, S. G. (2020) Eight weeks later — The unprecedented rise of 3D printing during the COVID-19 pandemic — A case study, lessons learned, and implications on the future of global decentralized manufacturing. *Applied Sciences*, 10(12), 4135.

Pikkarainen, M., Hyrkäs, E. & Martin, M. (2020) Success factors of demand-driven open innovation as a policy instrument in the case of the healthcare industry. *Journal of Open Innovation: Technology, Market, and Complexity*, 6(2), 1–16. doi: 10.3390/JOITMC6020039.

Polónia, D. F. & Gradim, A. C. (2021) Innovation and knowledge flows in health-care ecosystems: The Portuguese case. *The Electronic Journal of Knowledge Management*, 18(3), 374–391. Available at: https://academic-publishing.org/index.php/ejkm/article/view/2122/1949 (Accessed on 7 April 2021).

Sadr, M. & Granig, P. (2019) From ego to eco: What has VIENNO–the Vienna Innovation Model–got to do with it? In: *ISPIM Conference Proceedings*.

The International Society for Professional Innovation Management (ISPIM), pp. 1–8.

Salge, T. O. & Vera, A. (2009) Hospital innovativeness and organizational performance: Evidence from English public acute care. *Health Care Management Review*, 34(1), 54–67.

Sharar, S. R., Carrougher, G. J., Nakamura, D., Hoffman, H. G., Blough, D. K. & Patterson, D. R. (2007) Factors influencing the efficacy of virtual reality distraction analgesia during postburn physical therapy: Preliminary results from 3 ongoing studies. *Archives of Physical Medicine and Rehabilitation*, 88(12 Suppl 2): S43–S49.

Srai, J. S., Kumar, M., Graham, G., Phillips, W., Tooze, J., Ford, S., Beecher, P., Raj, B., Gregory, M., Tiwari, M. K., Ravi, B., Neely, A., Shankar, R., Charnley, F. & Tiwari, A. (2016) Distributed manufacturing: Scope, challenges and opportunities. *International Journal of Production Research*, 54(23), 6917–6935.

Chapter 1

Innovation in Healthcare — Beyond COVID-19 — Lessons Learned

Alan Cucknell, Laurence Weir, and Nigel Whittle FRSB

Plextek Services Limited, Great Chesterford, Saffron Walden, UK

hello@plextek.com

The COVID-19 pandemic is arguably the greatest healthcare crisis in the post-war era, causing huge disruption to global medical systems in addition to high rates of mortality and morbidity. But while it has caused dramatic upheaval worldwide, it has also led to a period of significant and positive innovation. This in turn has resulted in major advances in how healthcare is perceived and delivered. In the UK, we have seen fast-tracked digital adoption, centralised government support, and an urgency to find solutions in an entirely new social context. The subsequent paradigm shift in healthcare approach will have fundamental consequences for the industry.

In this chapter, we investigate how innovation driven by the pandemic is challenging conventional approaches to healthcare delivery and accelerating the development and adoption of new digital technologies and care models. We find that the blurring between medical industries, technologies and services has the potential to democratise healthcare provision, improving outcomes and experiences. But this future is far from certain and will depend on the attitudes of governments, regulators, and society towards a new digital healthcare paradigm.

1

1. Innovation Trends Necessitated by Crisis

A deadly combination of high infectivity, acute human population density and the severity of the illness, of which we had little prior knowledge or understanding, let alone treatments for, quickly made the emergence of COVID-19 a worldwide emergency.

While devastating, such significant upheaval often stimulates periods of profound change and innovation. In normal times, resistance to such change usually takes the form of existing power and commercial structures, which have vested interests in conservatism and dependency. But as we have seen with COVID-19, in times of crisis, the focus shifts as innovation becomes necessary for survival. In response to tremendous need, a unified, and often centralised, motivation to innovate arises. As Danish economist Ester Boserup said, 'necessity is the mother of invention'.[1]

In early 2020, governments around the world scrambled to secure the ability of their healthcare systems to sustain the onslaught of COVID-19. This was a challenging task as the crisis directly impacted the occupancy capacity of hospitals, the mental and physical health of staff, and delivery networks of healthcare supplies. Often the desired goals were not immediately achievable, such as when the demand for personal protective equipment (PPE), ventilators, oxygen and vaccines far exceeded available supply.

1.1. *A national scale threat — requiring central planning and logistics*

In ways not seen since the Second World War, governments have rolled out nationwide systems (or even international ones such as Covax) to centrally control aspects like COVID-19 testing or vaccine delivery. Fundamental to this has been central government's ability to requisition public buildings for such uses — and of course, lockdowns (and therefore, lots of empty units) made this easier — demonstrating that a centralised approach provides big advantages in situations where universal coverage is required. Governments have also had to make difficult judgement calls

---

[1] https://healthresearchfunding.org/ester-boserup-population-growth-theory-explained/.

as to how best to invest their economic strengths, either by funding long-term furlough schemes to protect jobs, to invest in technology to control the disease, or in long-term activities to develop effective countermeasures such as vaccines and drugs. While there are a variety of structural approaches taken internationally to deliver healthcare, in the case of the COVID-19 pandemic, centralised control was undoubtedly the best option due to the need for a rapid and large-scale response. It was a situation where market forces would simply not have had time to operate effectively.

This centralised approach, combined with the urgent medical supply needs at the beginning of the pandemic, triggered a wave of unusual healthcare innovation responses. For example, there was an initial drive to develop ventilators, which motivated players from other industries to develop and manufacture medical devices. In the UK, examples included domestic appliance manufacturer Dyson, aerospace manufacturer Rolls Royce and automotive manufacturer McLaren. For the most part, the ventilators themselves were not necessarily innovative — although there was an explosion of interest in different approaches, often from enthusiastic inventors rather than medical professionals — but what was innovative was the range of players that entered the market and the mechanisms through which they were motivated, coordinated and funded.

1.2. *A new enemy — requiring a new approach to testing and regulation*

With the advance of COVID-19 came the requirement to develop and deploy new tests, drugs and equipment quickly, while still adhering to the appropriate regulations. In the past, these processes have been much slower and more difficult. But the response to the pandemic demonstrated how different parts could be accelerated or even bypassed entirely.

Medically, condensing research and trials into weeks and months rather than years was incredibly challenging. In the normal course of pharmaceutical testing, contracts would not be finalised until all production processes had been defined and safety testing had been completed. But in this pandemic, governments invested huge sums of money in speculative activities. In the face of potentially catastrophic death rates, the urgent need for a vaccine greatly outweighed standard procedures, resulting in the most dramatic success story of the COVID-19 pandemic — the development, production and supply of several successful vaccines in an unprecedentedly short time.

This speed was only possible through parallel working at risk and because decisions to commission vaccine production without the usual evidence of efficacy were fully covered by government funding and support.

1.3. *An information problem — managing population engagement*

Alongside innovation, disinformation and the consumerisation of healthcare have been key components of the COVID-19 pandemic, along with the significant role played by the media and social media platforms. We've seen how vital accurate, transparent and consistent messaging is. Poorly done, it can be dangerously confusing — e.g. hydroxychloroquine being touted as a potential cure, but in later trials being shown to be ineffective. Done well, especially when supported by cultural norms and leadership behaviour, targeted communications have the potential to positively influence public response.

We've seen how very effective social media has been at spreading important centralised messages, but also unfounded speculation and conspiracy theories. It seems that disinformation is more easily spread when trust in public bodies is low. It is likely that in future crises, innovative means of spreading information, such as endorsement by YouTube influencers, will take the forefront over established mechanisms of information provision.

1.4. *A social virus — requiring remote healthcare*

With a need to minimise human contact to reduce virus transmission rates, we saw the rapid development and adoption of remote models for patient care. With face-to-face meetings no longer possible, many individuals (both practitioners and patients) have been forced to adapt to remote healthcare provision much faster than expected. For many, it has transformed their idea of what is possible. While there will remain certain cases where in-person meetings are necessary, this behaviour change forced upon us by the COVID-19 pandemic means many more people now appreciate that remote consultations can be more efficient, cost-effective and user-friendly.

Innovation, and new digital technologies, are at the core of enabling this shift, whether through smartphones and related wearables, or new advances in real-time patient monitoring and reporting. One example is the ZOE app in the UK, which allowed people to log daily symptoms and thereby centralise information gathering about the course of the pandemic.

In parallel, many nations are increasingly aware that moving long-term healthcare into the home setting, supported by remote technological advances, will be the most cost-effective way to address the future health-care needs of an ageing population. COVID-19, and the desperate urgency of keeping the most vulnerable safe, has only served to emphasise the advantages of this remote approach.

Despite its devastating social and economic consequences, there's no doubt that the COVID-19 pandemic has accelerated medical research and development — and in particular digital health technologies, which will result in fundamental changes to healthcare provision going forward.

2. The Digital Health Acceleration

Through the COVID-19 pandemic, we have seen that when healthcare systems are in crisis, and solutions are required that can be rapidly scaled to a national level, digital health technologies become an essential com-ponent of the ecosystem. In the unique arena presented by the pandemic, various technological solutions were embraced to improve the quality and accessibility of healthcare, while also reducing costs for both providers and end users. Many of these solutions were already in development pre-COVID-19, but the urgency of response required resulted in a dramatic speeding up of their roll-out and application. This has caused significant changes within the healthcare environment and will continue to influence future progress too.

Here we explore some of these key areas of digital health innovation, how they were leveraged in response to COVID-19, and what the health-care industry might look like in a post-pandemic world.

2.1. *Telehealth*

Telehealth — the delivery of healthcare from a distance — has become increasingly normalised over the course of the pandemic. With severe limitations on face-to-face meetings, in-person visits and hospital appointments, COVID-19 instantly impacted the usual doctor–patient relationship and interaction. New solutions were quickly needed. These were delivered via a range of related technologies — teleconferencing; remote monitoring devices; smartwatches, apps and wearables; and electronic connectivity — all of which contributed in integrated ways to enable some level of ongoing diagnosis, treatment, monitoring and patient care. These technologies are now here to stay, and as they become more integrated, will significantly influence the future of healthcare provision.

2.1.1. *Teleconferencing*

The most obvious manifestation of existing technology being used in new ways for the pandemic was teleconferencing, which allowed doctors, patients and medical professionals to continue to communicate effectively with each other. And it wasn't only at a local or national scale that telecommunication solutions were speedily adopted. With the severe COVID-19 wave in India in Spring 2021, some British doctors used tele-health systems to help alleviate the overloaded Indian healthcare systems by diagnosing patients remotely from the UK.

Even as society has begun to re-open, many are opting to remain with this remote setup. However, there are clear limitations to what can be done through this form of telehealth. Even as video conferencing becomes increasingly ubiquitous, there are issues with robust technology and reliable connectivity, as well as the fact that most nations still have a large and vulnerable section of society without access to the technology or not being comfortable yet to use it. Many patients still prefer face-to-face interactions and this is likely to be the case for a long while yet, particularly among the older generations. There are some impressive examples of health services using outreach programmes to take tele-health services to the vulnerable, such as by setting up doctor access points in homeless hostels and similar facilities — but much more needs to be done before we see complete engagement across all sectors of society.

In fact, it's not just the public who are reticent about telehealth, there are also issues with adoption rates among healthcare professionals. In the US in 2020, most remote healthcare consultations were conducted by telephone (and not video or web conference), as it was the format that healthcare practitioners were most comfortable with.

In addition, while improving patients' experience is usually touted as the main reason to use technology in healthcare, a recent survey[2] has highlighted that many doctors now fear working in 'call centres'. So as well as tackling any reticence to adopt new approaches, it is also going to be fundamental to reflect on how telehealth technology might impact the working environment for healthcare professionals and mitigate any negative effects accordingly.

Much of the reservation among medical professionals and the public towards telehealth is down to the fact that many of the current options have been rapidly deployed during the pandemic, often much quicker than originally intended. Sometimes execution has been effective; and at other times, limited.

Therefore, to learn from these lessons, now is the time to consider how to make more conscious and planned designs that will make telecommunications provision more efficient and effective, improve patient experience, enable secure management of confidential data, and benefit healthcare systems and medical professionals alike.

Further, while the COVID-19 pandemic has accelerated the move to digital delivery of healthcare, we must not forget that the growing treatment waiting lists at the end of the pandemic will require a variety of

---

[2]https://www.theguardian.com/society/2021/mar/28/gps-prefer-to-see-patients-face-to-face-says-uk-family-doctors-leader.

different solutions to support and care for patients. For many people, the current healthcare offering is hindered by issues around getting appointments, long waiting times in surgeries and poor communication. While these are generally accepted in the UK as *quid pro quo* for free access to the NHS at the point of delivery, in other countries the commercial nature of healthcare provision will necessitate faster improvements and continued innovation — developments that the UK can then learn from. Therefore, building on the experience of the pandemic, the goal going forward will be to work out what can and cannot be feasibly achieved through telecommunications platforms to improve the efficiency and effectiveness of healthcare provision.

2.1.2. *Remote monitoring*

Remote monitoring devices have the potential to provide a helpful early warning system, and a safe and easy way of delivering holistic ongoing patient care, particularly to those who are elderly, housebound or clinically vulnerable. For example, in January 2021 there was a scramble to buy personal blood oximeters as an early warning sign of deterioration in health due to COVID-19 infection. We also witnessed doctors in Israel using remote healthcare suitcases (combining a telecommunications solution and remote monitoring technologies) to follow up with COVID-19 patients recovering at home.[3]

However, generally patients will only engage with monitoring systems if there is a clear reward or benefit for them. So while the prospect of potentially coming out of lockdown sooner, or avoiding the need to self-isolate, motivated people to proactively collect, record and upload remote health data to their medical records during the COVID-19 pandemic, in more normal times, users would only tend to do this if there was minimal effort required, a specific incentive (e.g. a quicker/better care response), or it became fun (e.g. through gamification). Systems that build one or more of these reasons into the user experience are more likely to engage patients and secure better results.

---

[3] https://www.youtube.com/watch?v=MkpO5CIk6i8.

. It's also the case that while remote monitoring has strong merits in placing the emphasis on the patient to gather the data, it remains reliant on the input of experienced professionals to accurately analyse it. So even if patients can be actively engaged in collecting and submitting data, and it is combined and cross-referenced in a way that builds a complete profile of overall health, we will still need the expertise of medical practitioners to interpret the results of remote health systems.

Much has been learnt in this sphere over the course of the pandemic. Despite medical imaging being one of the most important technologies available for diagnosis and treatment, it is still hampered by several limitations. There's currently no single technology for the imaging of internal structures that is universally applicable to all tissues, has high resolution, is inexpensive, does not use ionising radiation and creates images in real time. Therefore, future innovation is likely to focus on overcoming these limitations and developing imaging systems that are universal, portable and low-cost, enabling them to be used remotely in ambulances and other out-of-hospital environments.

As the medical world turns its attention to long-term, mobile and even home-based imaging to shorten waiting lists and relieve hospital pressure for preventive screening and early detection of diseases, radar-based bio-sensing and imaging applications are likely to play an increasingly important role. The advantage of this approach includes the potentially low cost and small size of the required hardware, plus a wide application across fields as diverse as heart rate tracking, sleep monitoring and fall detection for the elderly, right across to screening of the cardiovascular system, breast cancer imaging and stroke detection.

The advancement of remote diagnosis will fall into three categories:

(1) Conditions able to be detected through ubiquitous personal items, like a smartphone camera. An example could be pictures of skin lesions or moles that could be analysed using an app or uploaded to a central database.
(2) Conditions where specially developed disposable devices have been created and must be analysed in a laboratory. Many of which can be shipped by post or couriered cheaply. An example of which could be getting DNA sequenced.

(3) Conditions which require large hospital-based equipment, such
as CT scanners, and unless these tests are transformed by new technology, they will continue to be done in hospitals or centralised
settings.

As technology improves, we also expect to see a greater application
of chatbots driven by artificial intelligence to conduct initial diagnosis,
with a human working collaboratively as a second stage in the process.
This integrated approach to health monitoring and measurement can also
provide more accurate alerts to anomalous physiological changes. These
then have the potential to identify deteriorating health or the onset of a
serious medical problem. This earlier diagnosis and treatment will generally be cheaper with a higher success rate.

2.1.3. *Smartwatches, apps and wearable devices*

In certain areas, medical technology was already making its way into the
home before the COVID-19 pandemic — through smartphone apps. For
example, apps which track and monitor the rehabilitation of patients, pre-
scribing specific exercises and routines tailored to their situation, all completed in the comfort of their homes.

Many wearable devices — such as fitness trackers, smartwatches and
smart rings — are now being designed with a primary function of personal
medical monitoring to measure a wide range of health-related functions.
and to assess overall health and fitness. These small lightweight devices,
which are worn on the body, can monitor vital signs such as temperature,
heart rate and breathing rate, and may also provide insights into the early
onset or progression of an illness.

A swell of interest in well-being — starting before the COVID-19
pandemic but directly enhanced through it — has led to a range of wellness apps linked to these consumer devices. This, of course, is matched
by increasing medical interest in the prevalence of lifestyle diseases.
So with the post-COVID-19 focus on healthy living as a preventative
action, the increase of wearable devices linked to health and well-being
apps is to be expected (both in terms of popularity and commercial
viability).

Smartwatches and other wearables have one big advantage over more standard medical remote monitoring devices. They tend to be worn daily. This means they offer the possibility to monitor a variety of biometric signals through routine use. Plus, their connectivity allows for the easy collection and transfer of health data with very little effort required from the user. Whereas in comparison, most people who have remote medical monitoring devices do not end up using them regularly, which makes it hard to identify an accurate base level. That's simply because, apart from people suffering from a particular serious medical issue such as diabetes or heart disease, the frequent measuring and recording of the health data do not seem relevant or important — as can be seen with the typical usage of home temperature or blood pressure monitors.

While most of the current smartwatches/wearables are not certified as medical devices given the complexity of measuring biometric signals accurately (e.g. measuring heart rate via wrist-worn solutions is generally accepted as being less precise than chest-worn monitors), their data are still extremely valuable. Especially because it's 'real world' input rather than a trial environment, which not only reduces the impact on both patient and study centres, but also potentially increases the validity of the data and allows access to a wider pool of patients.

The COVID-19 pandemic is clearly driving forward technological development in biometric tracking with several studies involving wearables being instigated during this period. With COVID-19 infection, cases can be mild or asymptomatic so it can be incredibly hard to control transmission. Data collected from wearable devices, coupled with analysis by algorithms, can detect early signs of COVID-19 infection. Meaning that:

(1) The data can provide individuals with information on whether to isolate or to seek medical treatment.
(2) The data can also enhance remote patient monitoring.
(3) Aggregate data taken from wearables can detect general patterns and trends within a population.
(4) Cumulative data can be used to identify geographical hotspots.

The difference between aggregate population studies and individual agency is also helpfully blurred by apps and wearables. Anonymised data can be very useful if created by a large enough dataset, especially if it is resistant to generating biases that can exist with such platforms, such as underrepresentation in the elderly. The key is to provide benefits to the individual, even if its greater utility is in the population level. For instance, the UK's ZOE app allowed you to book a COVID-19 test automatically if criteria are met when filling in daily symptoms.

There are multiple trials underway to examine whether wearables can help reduce COVID-19 infections in places ranging from care homes to the battlefield. Wearable technology for COVID-19 symptom analysis is being integrated with a range of materials, from rigid bangles, to smartwatches and very flexible smart clothing. Since these wearable devices in general measure standard physiological parameters, there is the clear possibility of their use for monitoring a whole range of other conditions, from seasonal flu to more chronic conditions such as Chronic Obstructive Pulmonary Disease (COPD).

However, a note of caution. The mobile app and wearable market can be alien to some members of the public, with the elderly and disabled populations being most left out of this technological advancement. Product designers must consider how all demographics within the population can access good monitoring, especially our most vulnerable, who if helped could potentially secure the greatest benefit from such devices. An example of this principle is the MonitorMe home telephone by Sanandco which integrates four vital signs monitors (temperature, heart rate, oxygen saturation and blood pressure) into an inclusively designed traditional phone handset which elderly consumers are familiar with.[4]

2.1.4. Electronic connectivity

As business gradually emerges from the constraints caused by the pandemic, we are seeing a significant surge in interest in development of connected smart technologies, particularly for the medical and healthcare sector. Many of these directly relate to the devices and systems previously mentioned.

---

[4] https://www.sanandco.com/monitorme/; the authors' company was involved in this development.

For example, during the pandemic, the UK's COVID-19 App was developed to detect contact between two users, automatically alerting one if the other had a positive test. While not always successful in its delivery and accuracy, the development of the app helpfully highlighted some serious challenges presented by this level of connectivity. Big questions were asked in terms of whether the UK Government should partner with corporate technology companies, like Google and Apple, to gain the data it needed to make the most effective application — and in future, the transference of patient data into corporate systems is a vulnerability that governments are likely to avoid. But in truth, it's also difficult to envision a future health event (outside another pandemic) that will require knowing exactly who you've been in contact with at the public health population level. However, we may start to see the use and development of these types of technologies at a community level in the future (e.g. to minimise the risk of seasonal flu for vulnerable sectors of the population).

At a personal level, connectivity between devices allows users to take greater responsibility for their healthcare and can potentially provide valuable insights into ongoing health issues without the need for frequent consultations with medical practitioners. Smart innovation in healthcare means not only developing and adopting new products and technologies for diagnosis and treatment, but also necessarily involves a greater degree of information exchange between devices and systems, which can enable better management of clinically relevant data.

At one end of the healthcare spectrum, a range of medical devices such as inhalers, insulin pens, blood pressure monitors, cardiac rhythm monitors, sleep therapy devices and the like are being developed as connected smart devices. These devices not only allow users to take increased responsibility for their health but through their connectivity, enable healthcare professionals to remotely monitor ongoing conditions. This facilitates observation and treatment that was previously only possible in a face-to-face medical setting (something that the COVID-19 pandemic has shown is truly advantageous).

Similarly, at the other end of the spectrum, there is rising interest in consumer wellness devices, with associated apps and platforms, to assess overall health and fitness (as mentioned in Section 2.1.3).

However, the routes for successful development of both these classes of products are rarely straightforward. While the lessons learned from the big surge in interest and adoption during the COVID-19 pandemic are helpful, companies still need to understand much more about how such devices will be used in 'the real world', what features are needed for a successful product, and how they can effectively collect meaningful data from the devices.

From a technical perspective, collection and analysis of data sourced from these systems will require secure communication systems and powerful algorithms for data processing. But most important will be an understanding of how this data can be collated, analysed and used to develop further insights of value to both the user and the developer. Can the data assist users to find increased value in the product and can they help them change behaviours or bring new benefits to their lifestyles? Companies need to consider the user interfaces and consumer enjoyment elements to ensure a continuation of service and real positive lifestyle change over time.

Connectivity, and a ubiquitous platform which collates the data, is key. The worst of all worlds would be having data on lots of different platforms, and the analysis of all these aspects of your health done separately. When you visit a doctor, they cross-reference all major aspects of your physical health (heart, BMI, diet, lungs, blood, urine sample, etc.), to come up with a diagnosis. Any digital platform needs to replicate this intelligent melding of all the separately collected data if it's going to do what's needed. As we'll see in the next section, cloud-based data collection hubs and machine learning/artificial intelligence systems are likely to play an increasingly important role.

2.2. *Artificial intelligence*

Even before COVID-19, artificial intelligence (AI) and machine learning (ML) technologies were beginning to have dramatic impacts on the healthcare industry — and with a new appreciation for the benefits of remote, efficient and flexible healthcare technologies acquired through the pandemic, this will only increase. There are already intriguing examples of how ML/AI systems can enable diagnoses from collected data even before the doctor, accurately predicting heart attacks or strokes, and potentially saving lives. Developments in the field are already being felt in sectors where current practices are slow, complex or require highly trained specialists. The current impact is likely to be dwarfed however by the future potential for increased accuracy in clinical diagnosis, prognosis and treatment.

Interestingly, some markets, such as China, had also already started to deploy AI-driven healthcare check-up booths (such as Ping An Good Doctor[5]) prior to the pandemic. This trend is likely to continue.

The most significant current area of activity is machine learning for medical imaging studies. The challenge for clinicians is to interpret the complexity of clinical images, which can be time-consuming, expensive, and prone to errors due to visual fatigue. With a huge backlog of patients, medical imaging and diagnosis departments would benefit hugely from machine learning to increase the speed and accuracy of their maxed-out working environments. Therefore, the potential for AI to help deal with increased screening demand due to a growing ageing population is huge.

Recent advances in deep learning show that computers can extract more information from images, with an increase in reliability and accuracy. Moreover, deep learning can be used to identify and extract novel features that would otherwise not be easily detectable by human viewers. In fact, a recent *Nature* article claimed that the AI analysis of lung cancer screening images can reduce mortality by 20–30% by being able to detect it earlier than a consultant viewing the images.[6]

AI also has a huge role to play in healthcare logistics. With supply chains and people tracking becoming more and more complex, AI systems have been deployed during the COVID-19 pandemic to improve the ability to keep things running efficiently. This was seen especially in commercial markets through the huge expansion of home delivery networks.

In a personal setting, AI is being used to track personal behaviour changes which could indicate health outcomes. A smartphone tracks its user most of the day, and therefore detects the level of movement activity,

---

[5] https://www.mobihealthnews.com/news/asia/ping-good-doctor-launches-commercial-operation-one-minute-clinics-china.
[6] https://www.nature.com/articles/d41586-020-03157-9.

places visited, hours asleep, and the products bought. The classic example of AI at work in this way is supermarkets being able to tell when regular shoppers are pregnant due to behavioural changes in purchases recorded via loyalty cards, and automatically shifting product marketing in response. So as AI systems become increasingly advanced in analysing data and correlating it with other factors such as geography and population-level studies, there is real potential for a smartphone — or the AI system powering it — to alert a user to a potentially serious illness before they are even aware of it themselves.

Mental health conditions are very difficult to diagnose accurately, often requiring analysis over an extended period and tending to be more closely linked to behaviour than any particular physical symptoms. Therefore, by tracking and analysing behaviour more closely, AI (as in the supermarket pregnancy example) could help alert users or healthcare professionals of potential mental health issues before they are otherwise revealed.

The rapid rise in health and behaviour data collected via smart devices means that personal data and population-level studies will also start to offer levels of insight into this area that previously would have taken years of research to attain. AI offers a way to access and share these insights for the benefit of all — because as big data matures and starts to cover decades of our lives, we will see fundamental changes in how this vast and valuable lifestyle data are used. This knowledge is currently owned and acted on by a very small number of extremely experienced workers in the field — but once an AI system can perform this role, the potential exists to democratise these data and their conclusions to the entire population.

In a commercial or hospital management setting, AI also has the potential to make health systems more efficient by having a greater oversight of the entire system and the ability to detect and eliminate the points of waste.

2.3. *Drones or unmanned aerial vehicles (UAVs)*

Since the beginning of the COVID-19 pandemic, the use of drones has hit record levels.

In China, then the world's most populous nation and where the COVID-19 outbreak first took hold, drones were used extensively for making medical deliveries to reduce in-person exposure, spraying disinfectant over large areas (using retrofitted agricultural drones), taking individuals' temperatures using thermal cameras and warning citizens to wear masks.

Similarly, in Spain, the police forces deployed drones to film streets and parks to help monitor the relaxation of lockdown rules. In North Carolina, Zipline was asked by Novant Health to begin delivering medical supplies, while Alphabet's Wing delivered food and OTC medical supplies in Virginia.

With drones, the main limiting factor regarding their use is not the technology *per se*, but the regulation. This limits the use of drones in built-up and uncontrolled areas, and prevents operation where visibility is degraded due to adverse weather conditions. It's right that these regulations exist — the consequences of unregulated flying of drones can be deadly serious. They can and do fall out of the sky. GPS systems are not as robust as we'd like and no one wants one to crash in a densely populated environment. Drones must also still be piloted, or at least have human pilot back-up and be flown within the line of sight of that pilot.

To address these issues, drones will need to be equipped with technology which will mitigate the risk of accidents to an acceptably low rate. In short, the route to secure fast roll-out of drones will be the creation of network of routes which minimise the risk to people and property if the drone was to fall.

As already shown by the use of drones during the COVID-19 pandemic, for items less than 10 kg (which covers a huge number of health-care supplies), the ability to transport these items without being constrained by the road/rail/sea network is going to be revolutionary. One thing for certain, the technology is already there. Radar technology, image analysis and drone flight technology are ready to be unleashed once the practicalities and regulations of flying have been fully addressed.

2.4. *Collaborative robotics*

One of the main groups of society that has suffered most during the COVID-19 pandemic has been the elderly, especially those who live alone or in managed-care environments. Solitude has a big impact on mental health. But with reduced human contact, their physical care has also been at risk.

In a post-COVID-19 world where social distancing may continue to be a serious consideration — especially around those most clinically vulnerable — collaboration with robots could be an immensely practical solution. For example, companion robots can be used to calm and reassure an elderly person, even one suffering from debilitating physical or mental health. A companion robot could also be helpful in monitoring for falls and calling for assistance when falls have occurred. There are also tasks for which robots, with their strength and capability for repetitive exact movements, are much better suited than humans.

Recent advances in technology have allowed robotic systems to be scaled down in size and cost from their industrial predecessors, allowing smaller robotic systems to play a more integrated role in environments such as life science laboratories. Totally automated solutions, with little human interaction, are still inherently inflexible and can be very expensive. With safety in mind, a preferred option has therefore been isolated islands of automation, perhaps functioning as a specific workstation within a laboratory, operating independently, but which can interact to a limited extent with nearby workers or caregivers.

In future, we might imagine a world in which humans and robots more actively collaborate on a specific project, working efficiently in tandem. Such robotic systems, commonly referred to as 'cobots', are now being designed to operate in proximity to humans, collaborate with them and move around independently in their shared workspace. They are still robots but freed from their constraints, and thanks to their small size and mobility, can be safely deployed in a range of environments.

Cobots must be equipped with safety sensors and software, and are often constructed of lightweight materials, with rounded edges, and with limitations on movement range, speed and force. Ideally, they slow down when a human worker is close to them, and if they bump into somebody, they stop immediately.

Further developments are likely to include improved user interfaces to allow for clear-cut interaction, and perhaps user-ID systems to allow interaction with specified individuals. Such systems will be easy to train in new tasks, thanks to machine learning processes whereby the cobot learns to complete a task through repeated interaction within a dynamic environment. As the technology develops, AI systems could then be introduced to predict actions and suggest improvements in procedures.

There is no doubt that many of the repetitive jobs performed by humans today will be done by robots in the future. But collaborative robotics demonstrates that such tasks can include highly interactive processes that provide a route to combining the skill that humans can bring with the capabilities of robots. This will allow activities to be conducted more effectively, while creating more challenging and rewarding jobs in the process. The healthcare sector, and in particular the increasing need to find efficient ways to care for an ageing population, is likely to be one of the main beneficiaries of such technological advances.

3. The Coming Digital Paradigm Shift — Industry Implications

We believe there are likely to be several key changes witnessed in the healthcare industry over the coming years as a direct result of the COVID-19 pandemic response — and in particular driven by the implications of the digital healthcare technologies outlined in the previous section.

3.1. *The blurring of healthcare*

Up until now, we have been used to a linear way of delivering healthcare in the UK — GPs/family doctors, referrals, A&E, hospital admissions and pharmacies. Going forward, we are likely to see healthcare provision cover a much wider spectrum than previously, incorporating social care, management of an ageing population, and much deeper, comprehensive support of mental health, well-being and healthy lifestyle choices.

Digital technologies are an enabler for patients, professionals and healthcare systems to leverage common data platforms. The ability in the future for healthcare-related data from multiple sources and services (e.g. hospital, GP, health club, smartphone, watch, etc. — even perhaps entertainment and social devices in time) to be accessed and analysed together has tremendous potential for preventative diagnosis and more holistic care. All of which will improve patient experiences, outcomes and reduce costs.

3.2. *Overlapping industries*

In future, a new healthcare provider might not come from the conventional medical sector. Instead, we will see elements of healthcare provision offered by tech companies previously focused on areas such as housing, insurance, tourism and lifestyle. That may be through consumer wellness devices that integrate with healthcare provision and monitoring (as outlined in Section 3.1), or by offering direct healthcare services, such as remote prescription processing and speedy delivery. With next-day delivery to most households in the country provided by companies like Amazon, people now expect convenience from all sectors and increasingly will not accept issues like in-person queuing at a pharmacy. It is worthy of note here that this disruption is not driven by technology alone, but by new business models inspired and enabled from adjacent industries.

3.3. *Healthcare disruptors*

Traditionally, a medicine-based business model required large companies (e.g. AstraZeneca, GSK, J&J, Bayer, Pfizer) that can invest in decades of chemical R&D, whereas modern MedTech disruptors can be lean start-ups with very short timeframes to delivery. However, the move to digital technologies in healthcare diagnostics, management and treatment — and the increasing availability and interoperability of these technologies — is dramatically lowering the barriers to entry. To what extent these opportunities will be maximised will depend on the continued appetite of regulators, harmonisation of standards and the degree of investment in research. While these changes in industry configuration were already happening, they have been significantly accelerated by the COVID-19 pandemic.

4. Conclusions — The Future of Healthcare

The COVID-19 pandemic has vastly accelerated the development and adoption of new healthcare devices and technology, arguably by 10–15 years. While many of these were already in the pipeline pre-COVID-19, the urgency of responding to the needs and challenges of a situation meant that the pandemic offered a whole new opportunity for rapid technological advancement and innovation.

The key factors that enabled this accelerated adoption were as follows:

- The necessity of action generated because of the scale and urgency of the COVID-19 pandemic.
- A centralised response which facilitated rapid planning and application of country-wide logistics, coordinated through national funding, support and a preparedness to take financial risks.
- The urgency for supplies and solutions generated an environment which positively encouraged unconventional or 'left-field' innovative answers, often provided by players from other industries.
- Unprecedented social restrictions with lockdowns, distancing and self-isolation required new ways of working and communicating, meaning remote, virtual solutions suddenly became invaluable.
- Much of the technology already existed, but the COVID-19 pandemic meant it was adopted much quicker and more comprehensively than it might have been (e.g. older generations adapting to video conferencing for medical appointments because there was no other choice).
- The pandemic created specific incentives for individuals to proactively monitor/collate/submit health data (e.g. ending lockdown sooner).
- While interest in using smart wearables to monitor health criteria predates COVID-19, the pandemic resulted in a surge (both among users and tech companies) because it naturally generated much more focus on well-being and tackling preventable lifestyle diseases (especially because of the health factors that made some individuals more vulnerable to suffering more severely with the virus, e.g. obesity).
- Because of the unique restrictions forced on society and the medical profession by the pandemic, the potential advantages of AI — such as

reduced workload for medical professionals, quicker, more accurate diagnosis, big data analysis and learning — became even more apparent, especially if given the right development and investment.

- Specific technologies such as drones were given an unprecedented opportunity to be tried and tested in real-life scenarios.
- The social challenges of the COVID-19 pandemic, especially isolation, showed how robotics could help in care settings.

Of course, the learning from the pandemic is not all rosy. Serious challenges with each type of digital innovation explored in this chapter have also become apparent. So much of this is simply down to the fact that much of the COVID-19-induced acceleration happened in the technical sphere, with an understandable focus on rapid roll-out and adoption, meaning that the business and social models still need to catch up. But even negative feedback can be valuable as it provides an opportunity for further development. So, accurate communication, especially in the social media sphere; secure and confidential management of data, with effective interpretation and analysis; avoidance of social alienation and inequality; incentivised and well-used remote monitoring information; digital training and outreach; sensible regulation and implementation — all these and more will need to be addressed going forward for the lessons of the pandemic to be truly built upon.

Above all, there is no doubt that the direction of healthcare provision will continue to change significantly in several ways over the coming years. We will see the blurring of healthcare with cross-industry delivery, new providers arising from different sectors, and a positive, proactive arena for modern MedTech disruptors to step into. While there's still much work to be done, and big hurdles to overcome, we believe that most of the new approaches outlined in this chapter will result in improved overall patient access to healthcare and facilitate better care of an ageing population in a post-COVID-19 environment.

So based on all we have learned so far, and the trends we perceive, this is what we imagine the future of healthcare will look like...

We believe we will start to see healthcare provision look more like the service Amazon offers to its customers than the current healthcare model. Drugs, supplements and specific lab tests will be delivered by courier or drones daily. Web portals will allow users to enter their details, and give permission for reasonably intrusive privacy invasions, in return for more efficiently delivered healthcare. If you have a symptom, you will be able to enter it onto your profile, to get an instant AI response directing you to either human referral or instant treatments. These will initially be completed through webchats, and then video conferencing. Telehealth will become a 'core' preventive service in supporting people with long-term chronic conditions. Home-based vital signs monitoring, enhanced point-of-care diagnostic systems with rapid turnaround, and app- and smartphone-based diagnostic systems will become the norm. There will also be improved early-stage access through remote and telehealth solutions, with chatbots increasingly used for initial diagnoses.

Data collected from your phone, smartwatches, and specific medical collection devices, like glucose monitors or blood oximeters, will be uploaded automatically and provide a broader picture of total health. An individual's entire medical and lifestyle history will be presented in a simple risk factor profile, which will instantly direct them to lifestyle improvements and well-being recommendations.

The healthcare system will be able to preferentially treat individuals who have these profiles, as they will have faster routes to delivery by using them. People who do not have this online health profile, or much-reduced data input, will be left with longer wait times for treatment, or further distances to travel. That said, we need to remain vigilant to avoid a digital divide between those patients with limited access to the new systems of healthcare delivery and those who are comfortable with such systems. Any new set-up must not disadvantage individuals who have no or inadequate digital access or skills; ensuring instead that capacity and resource is allocated to providing either alternative non-digital pathways or sufficient training and support. This is a complex problem but will need to be addressed if we wish to avoid increased inequality in access to healthcare, something that the NHS will rightly not tolerate.

Hospitals will still be needed to provide an A&E system, birthing centres, and specialised care for specific illnesses. But robots to deal with specific conditions or operations (like heart surgery) will be localised in only a few special units across the country. The speed, accuracy and reliability of these robots will outperform that of humans, and so it will be most efficient to bring patients to these robots, rather than having them distributed nationwide and not be fully utilised. Even if a human is required to operate the robot, they will not even need to be based in the same hospital, or country, or time zone (as in the example of the UK doctors treating Indian patients given at the start of the chapter).

Moving long-term healthcare into the home setting will also be increasingly acknowledged as the most cost-effective way to address the medical needs of an ageing population. The use of new telehealth and remote technologies will facilitate this, particularly through wearable tech for diagnosis and monitoring, teleconferencing for expert consultations, advanced fall detection systems, and the integration of appropriate technology into housing. However, we also need to ensure we don't totally eliminate the benefits of physical social interaction and community support, especially for older or more vulnerable individuals who are often already at risk of isolation.

One key question going forward is how will the funding model change? Will we see increases in funding from public or private sectors? The appetite for increasing public funding varies enormously from country to country — but one thing the COVID-19 pandemic has made very clear is that a centralised healthcare system makes the nationwide launch and delivery of new methods of healthcare provision significantly faster and easier. Trust, education, processes and partnerships can all be enablers or blockers and all too often we have seen good ideas fall down not because of the idea, but due to the way it is implemented.

Without a doubt, all these potential changes in healthcare provision will raise new issues to be overcome, some of which are impossible to predict. However, we believe that in a post-COVID-19 environment, where patient care will need to be as safe, effective and scalable as possible, the benefits of this wave of accelerated digital innovation will outweigh the negatives. Above all, the disruptive innovation generated in response to the COVID-19 crisis will continue to result in considerable advances in healthcare for the benefit of all. Embedding the lessons learned from the COVID-19 pandemic into our care and welfare systems will undoubtedly accelerate us towards exciting new technologies and innovative models of healthcare.

https://doi.org/10.1142/9781800614192_0002

Chapter 2

Hospital Innovation Management: An Assessment of Two State-Owned Portuguese Hospitals

Daniel Ferreira Polónia* and Adriana Coutinho Gradim†

Economics, Management, Industrial Engineering and Tourism Department, University of Aveiro, Campus Universitário de Santiago, Aveiro, Portugal

GovCOPP (Governance, Competitiveness and Public Policies) Research Unit, University of Aveiro, Campus Universitário de Santiago, Aveiro, Portugal

*dpolonia@ua.pt
†adrianacoutinho@ua.pt

This work aims to assess how innovation is managed by state-owned hospitals in Portugal. From an initial literature review, two research questions arise, the first addressing the current *status quo* on the management of innovation activities, and the second questioning if an innovation management system can bring value to the existing processes.

Based on the analysis of 10 interviews recorded in two institutions, how organisations manage innovation has been analysed.

The main conclusions point to the fact that hospitals seek to develop a manageable innovation strategy, creating incentives and structures to support innovation activities by their workers and parties involved in the innovation ecosystem. However, they still have difficulty in maintaining a steady and continuous innovation activity, and also have significant difficulties in monitoring and evaluating the impact of innovation activities, and associated results, on the organisation. Despite the existence of several indicators to monitor the innovation processes, due to the lack of resources, it is the *ex-ante* and the *ex-post* assessment of the innovation projects are often disregarded.

Considering the existing situation, and based on the evidence found, the implementation of an innovation management system could contribute to improve the performance of the organisation with regards to innovation. For that purpose, this work suggests the implementation of specific mechanisms to manage and monitor the innovation activities.

As for future research activities, they could extend the scope of the study to private and public hospitals to compare best practices and use a mixed-method approach to improve the scientific outcomes.

1. Introduction

In recent years, more active and demanding patients, as well as dynamic and open innovation ecosystems in healthcare, have promoted innovation to the top of the agenda of hospital managers. The rise of dynamic ecosystems in healthcare, and the need to manage the participating stakeholders, demands a new approach to the traditional 'command-and-control' management approach, replaced by the orchestration of the participants in the innovation process (Pikkarainen, Hyrkäs and Martin, 2020; Polónia and Gradim, 2021). To promote such an orchestration, hospitals need to change their approach to innovation, promoting a more dynamic approach that leverages the existing assets and promotes innovation and entrepreneurship among the involved stakeholders (Jelinek *et al.*, 2012; Cohen, 2013; Aanestad, Vassilakopoulou and Øvrelid, 2019).

Faced with challenging business conditions, that usually mean patients receiving increasingly sophisticated (and expensive) treatments, hospitals have been seeking alternative approaches to implement processes to manage their innovation environment (Caccia-Bava, Guimaraes and Guimaraes, 2009; Moreira, Gherman and Sousa, 2017). The establishment of a dynamic innovation ecosystem between different partners can lead to the creation of a unique environment, allowing for a better business performance and acting as a key driver for innovation (Suominen, Seppänen and Dedehayir, 2019; Polónia and Gradim, 2021).

This work studies how two state-owned (public) hospitals, located in the NUTS II Centro (PT) Region of Portugal (Keating, 2018), manage their innovation environment, with special emphasis on their strategic approach and implementation of innovation processes, as well as how innovation impact is internally leveraged and assessed.

The Portuguese national health system adopts a mixed funding model, with Bismarckian components (there are private hospitals and health insurance mechanisms available to the public) and Beveridgian components (the Portuguese state provides universal coverage, owning, financing and managing the 'National Health Service' and its institutions), with the majority of the Portuguese healthcare institutions being state-owned (public) hospitals (Simões, 2009).

The interest for innovation in the public sector has grown over the years (Arena *et al.*, 2020), and, in the healthcare sector, challenges such as increasing costs, the ageing population, intense competition and institutional pressures have led healthcare institutions in several countries to find solutions based on innovation (Yang, 2015). However, there is no unique definition of the term since innovation can be defined from various points of view (Herting, 2002; Gallouj, Merlin-Brogniart and Moursli-Provost, 2015; OECD/Eurostat, 2018).

For this study, Innovation in healthcare, definition as the introduction of new services, mechanisms, processes and technologies that allow healthcare professionals to focus on patient needs while enhancing quality, efficiency, safety and the outcomes of the clinical process (Wu and Hsieh, 2011; Arena *et al.*, 2020).

Innovation in healthcare includes analysing the range of cases that can be treated with the developed innovation while considering the risk for the patient (Russell, 1977). Although innovation has received more attention in recent years, it has always played a distinctive role in industries through time, acting as a pillar of global competitiveness and human progress. The healthcare sector is no exception and it is notorious that hospitals are trying to incorporate innovative routines and practices in their everyday activities to take advantage of clinical, organisational and technological opportunities (Salge and Vera, 2009; Schultz, Zippel-Schultz and Salomo, 2012).

The interest of hospitals to act, not only as 'mere consumers of novelty', but also as generators of innovative solutions, led to the need for developing proper mechanisms to manage innovation (Caccia-Bava, Guimaraes and Guimaraes, 2009; Salge and Vera, 2009; Arena *et al.*, 2020), with hospitals developing innovation strategies that aim to foster an innovation culture that is supported by a strategic leadership (Caccia-Bava, Guimaraes and Guimaraes, 2009; Labitzke, Svoboda and Schultz, 2014).

In the implementation of their innovation strategy, hospitals create structures for the development of these activities (Brewster *et al.*, 2015) and promote innovation-friendly human capital policies, along with infrastructures and resources for the practice of innovation (Salge and Vera, 2009; Sadeghifar *et al.*, 2014). Among the most relevant structures, the innovation business plan takes a leading role, allowing hospitals to adapt their strategy according to opportunities and risks (Anthony, Eyring and Gibson, 2006; Dixit, 2016) thus enabling the development and implementation of a strategic plan for innovation that generally improves the hospitals' performance, organisational development and competitiveness (Labitzke, Svoboda and Schultz, 2014).

Along the development of the strategic plan, those responsible for its implementation design the way research, development and innovation (RDI) processes are guided (Drury and Farhoomand, 1999). For example, a need for the development and implementation of idea selection and intellectual property valorization mechanisms was identified in the literature, which allow to define and assess the processes through indicators (Labitzke, Svoboda and Schultz, 2014; Hellström *et al.*, 2015).

Also, there is the need to foster the innovation ecosystem, its continual assessment and improvement, and identify funding mechanisms. It is believed that the successful management of internal and external partners involved in the innovation ecosystem can act as an enabler to foster innovation in hospitals (Adner and Kapoor, 2010; Colldén and Hellström, 2018).

To sustain a competitive advantage and have access to internal and external opportunities, hospitals are allocating more resources to the development of innovation activities (Yang *et al.*, 2017). The management of these activities relies on a structure that is responsible for coordinating, controling and evaluating innovation activities in the hospital (Labitzke, Svoboda and Schultz, 2014; de Kervasdoué, 2015) and also to ensure that innovations are incorporated into the daily practices of the organisation and valued accordingly (Schultz, Zippel-Schultz and Salomo, 2012; Labitzke, Svoboda and Schultz, 2014). Hospitals must then ensure the management of internal (e.g. human resources and strategic planning) as well as external opportunities (e.g. the management of partnerships) to develop a competitive advantage (Wu and Hsieh, 2011; Moreira, Gherman and Sousa, 2017).

Lastly, and of utmost importance, is the *ex-post* assessment of innovation results and impact in the organisations (Smith, 2005). The plan must include indicators and mechanisms that allow to formally and systematically assess the impact of innovation and its results (Bernardo, Valls and Aparicio, 2011; Brewster *et al.*, 2015). The development of a system to assess these issues can help to continuously improve the processes and define innovation opportunities that are relevant for the sustainability of the hospital (Bugge, Bloch and Mortensen, 2011; Wu and Hsieh, 2011; Improta *et al.*, 2012).

Since there is still limited research regarding the relationship between innovation mechanisms and their practice in hospitals (Yang *et al.*, 2017), this study aims to answer the following research questions:

RQ1: How are Portuguese state-owned hospitals managing their innovation activities, considering their structure and strategy, RDI processes, innovation enablers and assessment of innovation impact and results in the institutions?

RQ2: How are innovation activities managed and monitored in hospitals and what role can an innovation management system play?

Studies regarding hospital innovation are in need to help to understand how they evolve and adapt to the challenges of the surrounding environment (Yang, 2015). Answering these two research questions, this work aims to contribute to the literature by providing a case study of hospitals in the NUTS II Centro (PT) Region of Portugal that are in the phase of developing and/or implementing innovation management processes.

2. Methods

In the development of this study, a qualitative approach was used (Brewster *et al.*, 2015) through presential semi-structured interviews. The study was designed to determine how the selected hospitals are managing their innovation activities.

The inclusion of two hospitals, one of medium dimension and the other of large dimension, enables the comparison between the available resources and how efficiently innovation is managed. Since both hospitals present a similar innovation strategy and structure, the results from the study are generalised, as can be seen in the following section. In each hospital, five people involved in innovation projects and their management were selected for semi-structured interviews to ensure consistency (Brewster *et al.*, 2015).

For this work, the interviewees were selected by a senior executive in each institution. Participants were questioned about the innovation management processes adopted in the institution, including its development, implementation, and assessment. Moreover, according to the background and experience of each participant, the interviews focused on their area of expertise. For example, the people involved in the RDI unit of one of the hospitals were asked about the processes adopted there and how they impact the organisation; financial managers were asked about the implementation of mechanisms to assess the financial and operational impact of innovation in the hospital and hospital managers were asked about the vision regarding the role of innovation in the institution.

To guide the semi-structured interviews, a set of questions were adapted from the IMP³ROVE and the Innovation Scoring from COTEC questionnaires (COTEC, 2020; IMP³ROVE Academy, 2020). Even though these base questionnaires are strongly focused on the industrial sector, they were adapted to the healthcare sector, through a dynamic revision and adaptation process with the interviewees, thus enabling a heuristic understanding of hospital innovation management in a broader sense. Also, the questions were aligned with the literature's best practices (Salge and Vera, 2009; Weng *et al.*, 2011; Wu and Hsieh, 2011; Jacobs *et al.*, 2017).

The final version of the questionnaire focused on a diverse range of questions related to innovation management such as organisational strategy and structures, innovation processes, innovation enablers, innovation impact on the organisation and innovation results assessment.

A template for the report of each interview was created to include information according to the interview script. The first section focuses on a technical sheet that includes the name of the organisation, interviewee, interviewers, and date. The following section contains the healthcare institution's main data such as name, creation date, address and contact information, together with an analysis of the internal and external context of the organisation. Then there is the transcription of the interview which includes information regarding the identification of critical areas of the strategy, resources, processes, best practices and funding opportunities of the organisation. Lastly, the conclusions for each interview are addressed followed by suggestions for improvement.

Moreover, for each hospital, a general report was produced considering the interviews from each institution. This report allowed to compare answers, identify best practices and issues that need further improvement and that are mentioned by more than one person.

3. Results

For this study, a total of 10 people were interviewed. Interviewees from the two hospitals represented a wide range of positions, including managers, clinicians, nurses, academics and members of the unit of RDI as well as from the Board of Administration (Table 1). This variety of roles allowed to achieve a heuristic vision of the institutions and how the innovation management is perceived in the different services.

The interviews lasted, on average, one hour and both interviewers took notes during the interviews to compare them while writing the transcription of each interview. The notes taken by both interviewers allowed to guarantee the quality of the collected information. After the transcription, each report was sent to the interviewee so that they could assess the need to add further information, which did not happen in any of the cases.

Table 1.   Roles of interviewed persons.

Project manager	2
Hospital manager	2
Head of clinical service	2
Head nurse	1
Assistant to clinical management	1
Chairman of the board	1
Member of the board	1
Total	10

The results from the interviews were then analysed according to the structure of the interview script, namely divided into organisation structure, organisation strategy, RDI process, innovation enablers, innovation impact on the organisation and innovation results assessment.

3.1. *Organisation strategy*

To evaluate the degree of innovativeness in hospitals' strategy, participants were asked about how they monitor internal and external environments and the use of innovative technologies, the vision of innovation, the culture of innovation and the degree to which the employees are involved in innovation activities.

From this set of questions, it was possible to conclude that both hospitals define a yearly strategic plan which aims, as mentioned by one participant, to

> *Qualify[ing] services for development and innovation activities, in order to align services for the best performance.*

However, even though there are monitoring mechanisms in the strategic plan, they tend to be reactive, and the innovation strategy depends on the elements of each service of the institution. Considering that there are services more motivated to implement innovation projects and activities than others, this leads to a misalignment of the strategy in the institution.

Also, it is notorious that top management fosters a culture of innovation, by promoting the involvement of the employees in the innovation activities. This is a positive aspect that needs to be enhanced, since it is argued that a leadership that fosters an innovation culture can improve the service provided by its institution (Herting, 2002; Dobrzykowski, Callaway and Vonderembse, 2015).

However, according to the individual characteristics of the leadership members (Kimberly and Evanisko, 1981), which cannot be ignored, the fostering and improvement of the innovation culture will always be dependent on the individual:

> *The board changes every three years. Depending on the ambitions of the person who is nominated, the previous work can be compromised.*

At the same time, these two state-owned hospitals, like the others of the same type, are dependent on a central management system (National Health Service, 2020, 2021).

In Beveridgian systems, the policies and innovation guidelines defined by the government tend to influence the degree of innovativeness in hospitals (Kutzin, 2011). Analysing the documents related to the establishment of a health strategy and governance model in Portugal, it was found that there are no specific guidelines related to innovation practices. Nevertheless, a Clinical Research and Biomedical Innovation Agency was created with the objective of coordinating and stimulating innovation in healthcare and academic institutions (AICIB, 2021). However, hospitals still tend to have self-managed innovation processes (National Health Service; Health Directorate General, 2017).

Also, it was found that the motivation of the employees to participate in innovation activities tends to be different, according to the capacity of the hospital (Herting, 2002). Larger hospitals tend to innovate more and can define non-financial and financial rewards more easily than smaller hospitals (Blank and Valdmanis, 2015).

The integration of a clinical academic centre including hospitals and universities of the region was also found a valuable aspect. The coordination of activities between the organisations allows to access more resources for the practice of innovation activities and enter more innovation projects and funding opportunities.

3.2. *Organisational structure*

The way the institution is structured influences its behaviour (Kimberly and Evanisko, 1981). In this section, the focus was to find how organisations are structured for innovation activities. The participants were asked about the flexibility of the business plan, the infrastructures available for innovation, the human capital policies and how the institution fosters employees' creativity, as well as the organisational and technical skills available to promote innovation.

It was in this section that most divergences were found. Although both institutions have a strategic plan regarding innovation, there are no formal mechanisms implemented to manage it. This is alarming since in the literature, although it is mentioned that the organisational structure by itself does not influence innovation, there are claims that governance mechanisms tend to have a positive effect on innovation (Yang *et al.*, 2017). Even though it was mentioned that the people in the institution always try to do better and innovate, the lack of resources to innovate is significant:

> *Due to the lack of resources to implement mechanisms to manage innovation, the projects developed are mainly motivated by an individual desire of the person who proposes the project. For these, external funding needs to be identified and the management of the project as well as its assessment tends to be delayed.*

Although the leaderships of both hospitals develop human capital policies to promote the creativity of the employees, the development of technical and organisational skills for innovation tends to have an individualistic character, based on each individual's aim. This constitutes a problem since the individual objectives can be misaligned with institutional ones. Managerial systems need to be reinforced, with planning and control and human resources management systems that enable proper monitoring systems (Lega, 2009).

3.3. *Research, development and the innovation process*

In this section, participants were asked about the process of idea evaluation, project selection, intellectual property management, the use of key performance indicators (KPIs) and the rewards for those who engage in innovative projects. This is important since, in the current paradigm, hospitals need to change their processes and try to implement documented and systematic procedures (Ghasemi, Ghadiri Nejad and Bagzibagli, 2017).

Confirming what was previously found in this study, neither of the institutions has a global mechanism to manage innovation.

As mentioned by one participant:

> *Most of the innovation projects start based on an individual desire to innovate.*

It was found that each department tries to implement its own mechanism to manage innovation. This leads to a lack of integration in the institution, which can reduce the potential to develop and sustain new practices (Caccia-Bava, Guimaraes and Guimaraes, 2009; Brewster *et al.*, 2015). Also, it was found that, by implementing different mechanisms, the departments try to define and use KPIs. However, due to the reduced number of resources, the monitoring of the project and its *ex-ante* and *ex-post* evaluation tends to be neglected.

Moreover, most of the projects do not have mechanisms that enable the protection of the Intellectual Property (IP) generated. This happens since, in most of the cases, hospitals enter innovation projects with organisations that create and protect most of the intellectual property thus ensuring a vivid discussion regarding the accessibility to data and their ownership. So, hospitals tend to have a secondary role along the process which leads them to contractually void the rights to claim any contribution in the process (Sorbie *et al.*, 2021).

Considering the nature of hospitals as service providers, most of them do not prioritise innovation as a tool to improve the performance of the organisation or to create services and products that can add value to the institution (Labitzke, Svoboda and Schultz, 2014). This also leads to the lack of best practices regarding innovation from collaborations between institutions (Duarte, Goodson and Dougherty, 2014; van Veghel, Marteijn and de Mol, 2016).

Although the process to manage innovation is difficult to define and measure, it was found that both institutions always try to define financial and non-financial rewards for those involved in the projects. For example, one hospital finances the best articles and their publication every year and the other finances advanced training for its staff.

3.4. *Innovation enablers*

Due to the known difficulty of Portuguese hospitals to innovate (Dias and Escoval, 2012, 2014; Health Cluster Portugal, 2019), this section allowed to identify how these institutions are managing this challenge. For this reason, participants were asked about the involvement of the institution in the surrounding ecosystem, how they finance innovation projects, how they manage the acquired knowledge, and how they evaluate the activities performed.

Due to the changes in the healthcare sector, the importance of successfully engaging in cooperative networks of actors for value co-creation is known (Dobrzykowski, Callaway and Vonderembse, 2015; Gallouj, Merlin-Brogniart and Moursli-Provost, 2015). For both hospitals, the involvement in an innovation ecosystem with different entities from the public and private sectors was identified, which implies a complex dynamic among participants (Gallouj, Merlin-Brogniart and Moursli-Provost, 2015), as well as its proper management.

However, a lack of resources to implement a formal mechanism to manage partnerships was identified. Nevertheless, one of the hospitals has successfully entered in international networks that allows the institution to integrate projects at a European level, with access to more funding opportunities. As found in the literature 'the more complex innovations in external relations involve healthcare networks' (Djellal and Gallouj, 2007).

Regarding the financial opportunities for innovation, in neither of the two hospitals was there a formal budget defined for this type of activities. The institutions, proactively, identify external funding sources and projects are mainly financed by European funds as Horizon2020 and European Regional Development Funds (European Commission, 2020; Portugal 2020, 2020).

As mentioned by participants of both hospitals:

> *We must proactively seek financing opportunities for innovation, since there is not a clear budget allocated for this type of activities.*

Regarding the knowledge management process, it was found that the knowledge acquired from the participation in innovation projects tends to be formally managed. Since it is a co-creation among different actors, knowledge is the product of their interactions. As so, the implementation of knowledge-sharing routines can allow the hospital to 'produce complementary capabilities' (Schultz, Zippel-Schultz and Salomo, 2012; Dobrzykowski, Callaway and Vonderembse, 2015).

However, in neither of the two hospitals was a systematic knowledge management and sharing mechanism identified. Moreover, it was also found that the way people in the institution react to innovation can positively or negatively impact the sharing of knowledge, as found in the literature (Zweifel, 1995; Leal-Rodríguez *et al.*, 2013). As one of the participants mentioned:

> *We can define the strategies and implement them. However, if people decide to not share knowledge, it can affect the strategies and their effects.*

Also, although it is available as a systematic process to evaluate innovation activities, it is not structured or globally defined. However, it is argued in the literature that the development and implementation of a systematic process to manage innovation can positively impact an institution (Zweifel, 1995; Yang *et al.*, 2017).

3.5. *Innovation impact on the organisation*

This section, regarding the evaluation of the impact of innovation on the organisation, asked participants about the impact of innovation activities on the acquisition of new skills and competences, on the institution's reputation and image and on economic, social, environmental and financial sustainability.

The analysis of the impact of the innovation must consider measuring, reporting and comparing the outcomes (Jacobs *et al.*, 2017). The use of indicators can then help to monitor and evaluate innovation (Yang *et al.*, 2017). From the interviews and the questionnaire, it was identified that although hospitals define KPIs, they tend not to focus on the innovation impact, and that the lack of resources (people, time, know-how) does not allow for the development and implementation of a systematic evaluation process:

> *How can we allocate resources to manage innovation if we have difficulties and lack of resources to manage the daily basic activities?*

Regarding the acquisition of new skills and competences, the participants of both institutions highlighted the existence of financial and non-financial rewards systems, which is considered a motivation factor to engage in innovation activities (Schultz, Zippel-Schultz and Salomo, 2012).

3.6. *Innovation results assessment*

The last section of the interview asked participants about the existence of a mechanism that allows to evaluate *ex-ante* and *ex-post* innovation process, the investment in human resources for innovation and the benchmarking of value creation.

As previously demonstrated, there is a generic lack of resources and infrastructures to develop and implement systematic monitoring mechanisms to assess the innovation results. Despite the non-existence of a structured and systematic process that allows to assess the innovation results in either of the hospitals, it was found that in one of the hospitals a unit for RDI exists, that

> *Seeks to evaluate what the result is at the end of the project to understand the impact that the use of resources had on the organization.*

Considering that this process is not formally implemented and systematised throughout the institution, it amounts to a loss in terms of knowledge and gains from the RDI activities developed.

Although there is no formal process, in terms of human resources management, it was found that both hospitals try to follow those involved in the projects to reward them for the participation. The need to assess the results from innovation is real and hospitals must try to allocate human resources who are able to manage innovation and diffuse its results (Drury and Farhoomand, 1999; Jacobs *et al.*, 2017).

4. Discussion

To answer the first research question, it was found that the RDI unit of one of the hospitals develops and implements an innovation management process to all the institutions. Also, it was clearly mentioned that neither of the two institutions tends to have an innovation management strategy that is developed, implemented and assessed. This happens because, despite seeking to develop this innovative strategy, there is a lack of human and financial resources, as well as infrastructures that allow the implementation of systematic processes for the development, monitoring and management of projects of this nature.

Regarding the second research question, the management of innovation in hospitals is very important since the effective hospital innovation management tends to positively affect its performance. However, the determinants of hospital innovation are still not clear (Yang, 2015).

The management of innovation activities allows to assess what is being done right while identifying areas for improvement. The implementation of an innovation management process can help hospitals to be integrated in international networks, enabling the participation in European projects and access to other funding opportunities.

To conclude, it was found that hospitals seek to develop an innovation strategy to manage innovation in their institutions. However, it was identified that each department tends to have its own strategic plan, which leads to a dispersion of innovation efforts and management. The integration and alignment of the processes can benefit the institutions by helping innovation become a sustainable activity (Brewster *et al.*, 2015).

The development and implementation of innovation management mechanisms need to align elements from different departments, managers need to have the ability to manage risks and opportunities, the process needs to be clearly communicated as well as its progression and a management team needs to be defined in order to quickly respond to any issue that may arise (Caccia-Bava, Guimaraes and Guimaraes, 2009; Li *et al.*, 2017).

Also, it was assessed that there is no specific funding defined for RDI activities. For the development of innovation activities, leaders have sought to develop mechanisms to motivate their employees' participation in projects. There is proactivity on the part of organisations in the search for alternative sources of financing (Horizon2020 and ERDF are the most referenced).

Despite the definition of KPIs, there is still difficulty in monitoring and evaluating the impact of innovation activities on an organisation, as well as their results. It should be noted that, despite the difficulties experienced, hospitals have sought to foster RDI projects as well as the implementation of innovation management mechanisms.

4.1. *Implications for practice and research*

Considering the good practices identified, it is suggested that the organisations interviewed can implement the following road map.

It is observed that mainly due to the lack of resources (people, time, financing, infrastructure, knowledge) hospitals are unable to implement mechanisms for the effective management of their innovation practices.

Aligned with what was found in the literature and discussed with the participants in this study, first, it is suggested that hospitals should seek to allocate resources dedicated exclusively to innovation management in the organisation, coordinating an innovation management team, with roles and responsibilities clearly defined. The top management should encourage its employees to take risks and question existing processes (Herting, 2002), and leadership must also foster an innovation culture that can act as an enabler for the innovation practice (Weng, Huang and Lin, 2013).

With these basic processes enabled, it is possible to implement specific mechanisms to manage and monitor the following: the surrounding environment (strategic intelligence), the generation of ideas, partnerships, the intellectual property and the KPIs aligned with the global innovation strategy of the organisation (Schultz, Zippel-Schultz and Salomo, 2012). This can be done by adapting the ISO 56000 family of standards on innovation management (Tidd, 2021).

Currently, due to social, financial, political and even environmental changes, hospitals the world over are facing difficulties. These leads to the need to be more innovative in order to provide the best service (Lega, 2009). Moreover, with the COVID-19 pandemic, the need to establish collaborative relationships that foster innovation to offer better healthcare services is placing significant challenges before hospital managers (Chesbrough, 2020; Yang *et al.*, 2020).

For this reason, the implementation of mechanisms to manage and monitor innovation in hospitals is necessary (Ghasemi, Ghadiri Nejad and Bagzibagli, 2017). The main topics to help hospitals create an innovation management process are shown in Figure 1.

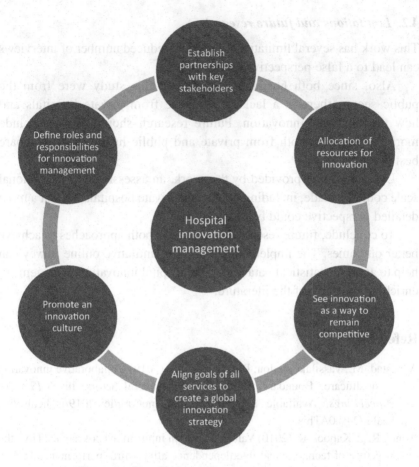

Figure 1.   Hospital innovation management process.

However, the literature regarding hospital innovation management is scarce. There is a need not only to develop a more theoretical background but also to develop studies relating to how hospitals are monitoring and assessing innovation (Jacobs *et al.*, 2017).

This study aims to offer the opportunity for researchers to explore hospital innovation management in different countries and healthcare sectors (public and private). The comparison between different countries and contexts and its diffusion can help not only to broaden the theory, but also to achieve best practices relating to innovation management in hospitals.

4.2. *Limitations and future research*

This work has several limitations. First, the reduced number of interviews can lead to a false perspective of the reality.

Also, since both hospitals included in this study were from the public sector, there is a lack of evidence from private hospitals and how they manage innovation. Future research should aim to include more participants, both from private and public hospitals, to compare best practices.

Using the input provided by this work, an assessment at the national scale could be made, including public and private hospitals, so that a more detailed perspective could be obtained.

To conclude, future researchers could use both approaches to achieve better outcomes. The implementation of a quantitative online survey can help to achieve statistical data regarding hospital innovation management, enriching the body of the literature.

References

Aanestad, M., Vassilakopoulou, P. & Øvrelid, E. (2019) Collaborative innovation in healthcare: Boundary resources for peripheral actors. In: *ICIS 2019 Proceedings*. Available at: https://aisel.aisnet.org/icis2019/is_health/is_health/24%0AThis.

Adner, R. & Kapoor, R. (2010) Value creation in innovation ecosystems: How the structure of technological interdependence affects firm performance in new technology generations. *Strategic Management Journal*, 31, 306–333.

AICIB (2021) *Agência De Investigação Clínica E Inovação Biomédica*. Available at: https://aicib.pt/ (Accessed on 16 March 2021).

Anthony, S. D., Eyring, M. & Gibson, L. (2006) Mapping your innovation strategy. *Harvard Business Review*, pp. 104–113. Available at: http://search.epnet.com/login.aspx?direct=true&db=buh&an=20454028.

Arena, C., *et al.* (2020) The adoption of e-Health in public hospitals. Unfolding the gender dimension of TMT and line managers. *Public Management Review*, 1–27. doi: 10.1080/14719037.2020.1775280.

Bernardo, M., Valls, J. & Aparicio, P. (2011) Organisational innovations in Catalan hospitals: The case of telemedicine. *International Journal of Healthcare Technology and Management*, 12(3–4), 307–320. doi: 10.1504/IJHTM.2011.040481.

Blank, J. L. T. & Valdmanis, V. G. (2015) Technology diffusion in hospitals: A log odds random effects regression model. *International Journal of Health Planning and Management*, 30(3), 246–259. doi: 10.1002/hpm. 2232.

Brewster, A. L., *et al.* (2015) Integrating new practices: A qualitative study of how hospital innovations become routine. *Implementation Science*, 10(1), 1–12. doi: 10.1186/s13012-015-0357-3.

Bugge, M. M., Bloch, C. & Mortensen, P. S. (2011) *Measuring Public Innovation in the Nordic Countries: Copenhagen Manual*, Nordisk institutt for studier av innovasjon, forskning og utdanning.

Caccia-Bava, M. C., Guimaraes, V. C. K. & Guimaraes, T. (2009) Testing some major determinants for hospital innovation success. *International Journal of Health Care Quality Assurance*, 22(5), 454–470. doi: 10.1108/ 09526860910975571.

Chesbrough, H. (2020) To recover faster from COVID-19, open up: Managerial implications from an open innovation perspective. *Industrial Marketing Management*. doi: 10.1016/j.indmarman.2020.04.010.

Cohen, E. (2013) Accelerating digital health innovation: Analyzing opportunities in the healthcare innovation ecosystem. Massachusetts Institute of Technology.

Colldén, C. & Hellström, A. (2018) Value-based healthcare translated: A complementary view of implementation. *BMC Health Services Research*, 18(1), 1–11. doi: 10.1186/s12913-018-3488-9.

COTEC (2020) *Innovation Scoring*. Available at: https://www.innovationscoring.pt/ (Accessed on 8 April 2020).

de Kervasdoué, J. (2015) Innovation et organisation hospitalière. *Presse Medicale*, 44(4), 381–382. doi: 10.1016/j.lpm.2015.01.002.

Dias, C. & Escoval, A. (2012) The open nature of innovation in the hospital sector: The role of external collaboration networks. *Health Policy and Technology*, 1(4), 181–186. doi: 10.1016/j.hlpt.2012.10.002.

Dias, C. & Escoval, A. (2014) Hospitals as learning organizations: Fostering innovation through interactive learning. *Quality Management Health Care Journal*, 1–8. doi: 10.1097/qmh.0000000000000046.

Dixit, S. K. (2016) Strategic management in hospitals — Theory and practice: Orthopedic and spine services. *International Journal of Healthcare Management*, 9(3), 181–189. doi: 10.1179/2047971915Y.0000000004.

Djellal, F. & Gallouj, F. (2007) Innovation in hospitals: A survey of the literature. *European Journal of Health Economics*, 8(3), 181–193. doi: 10.1007/ s10198-006-0016-3.

Dobrzykowski, D. D., Callaway, S. K. & Vonderembse, M. A. (2015) Examining pathways from innovation orientation to patient satisfaction: A relational view of healthcare delivery. *Decision Sciences*, 46(5), 863–899. doi: 10.1111/deci.12161.

Drury, D. H. & Farhoomand, A. (1999) Innovation diffusion and implementation. *International Journal of Innovation Management*, 03(02), 133–157. doi: 10.1142/s1363919699000074.

Duarte, N. T., Goodson, J. R. and Dougherty, T. M. P. (2014) Managing innovation in hospitals and health systems: Lessons from the malcolm Baldrige National Quality Award Winners. *International Journal of Healthcare Management*, 7(1), 21–34. doi: 10.1179/2047971913Y.0000000052.

European Commission (2020) *Horizon 2020 | The EU Framework Programme for Research and Innovation*. Available at: https://ec.europa.eu/programmes/horizon2020/en (Accessed on 9 April 2020).

Gallouj, F., Merlin-Brogniart, C. & Moursli-Provost, A. C. (2015) Public-private partnerships in hospital innovation: What lessons for hospital management? HAL. doi: 10.4337/9781781002667.00019.

Ghasemi, M., Ghadiri Nejad, M. & Bagzibagli, K. (2017) Knowledge management orientation: An innovative perspective to hospital management. *Iranian Journal of Public Health*, 46(12), 1639–1645.

Health Cluster Portugal (2019) *HCP's X Annual Conference | 'Unveiling the Future of Health and Care' — Health Cluster Portugal*. Available at: http://healthportugal.com/noticias/x-conferencia-anual-do-hcp-unveiling-the-future-of (Accessed on 2 January 2020).

Health National Service; General Health Direction (2017) *2020 Governance Model*. Available at: https://www.dgs.pt/documentos-e-publicacoes/modelo-de-governacao-a-2020-do-plano-nacional-de-saude-e-programas-de-saude-prioritarios-pdf.aspx (Accessed on 14 April 2020).

Hellström, A. *et al.* (2015) Adopting a management innovation in a professional organization: The case of improvement knowledge in healthcare. *Business Process Management Journal*, 21(5), 1186–1203. doi: 10.1108/BPMJ-05-2014-0041.

Herting, S. R. (2002) Trust correlated with innovation adoption in hospital. *The Innovation Journal: The Public Sector Innovation Journal*, 7(2), 1–29.

IMP³ROVE Academy (2020) *IMP³ROVE Assessment*. Available at: https://www.imp3rove.de (Accessed on 8 April 2020).

Improta, G., *et al.* (2012) An innovative contribution to health technology assessment. *Studies in Computational Intelligence*, 431, 127–131. doi: 10.1007/978-3-642-30732-4-16.

Jacobs, M., *et al.* (2017) What is the impact of innovation on output in healthcare with a special focus on treatment innovations in radiotherapy? A literature review. *British Journal of Radiology*, 90(1079). doi: 10.1259/bjr.20170251.

Jelinek, M., *et al.* (2012) 21st-century R&D. *Research Technology Management*, 55(1), 16–26. doi: 10.5437/08956308X5501011.

Keating, M. (2018) *Regions in the European Union. Nomenclature of Territorial Units for Statistics — NUTS 2016/EU-28*. Publications Office of the European Union, Luxembourg. doi: 10.2785/475524.

Kimberly, J. R. & Evanisko, M. J. (1981) Organizational innovation: The influence of individual, organizational, and contextual factors on hospital adoption of technological and administrative innovations. *Academy of Management Journal*, 24(4), 689–713. doi: 10.2307/256170.

Kutzin, J. (2011) Bismarck vs. Beveridge: Is there increasing convergence between health financing systems? Paris. Available at: https://www.oecd.org/gov/budgeting/49095378.pdf.

Labitzke, G., Svoboda, S. & Schultz, C. (2014) The role of dedicated innovation functions for innovation process control and performance — an empirical study among hospitals. *Creativity and Innovation Management*, 23(3), 235–251. doi: 10.1111/caim.12068.

Leal-Rodríguez, A. L., *et al.* (2013) Knowledge management, relational learning, and the effectiveness of innovation outcomes. *The Electronic Journal of Knowledge Management*, 11(1), 62–71. doi: 10.1080/02642069.2013.815735.

Lega, F. (2009) Strategic, organisational and managerial issues related to innovation, entrepreneurship and intrapreneurship in the hospital context: Remarks from the Italian experience. *Journal of Management & Marketing in Healthcare*, 2(1), 77–93. doi: 10.1179/mmh.2009.2.1.77.

Li, X., *et al.* (2017) Exploring the innovation modes and evolution of the cloud-based service using the activity theory on the basis of big data. *Cluster Computing*, 21(1), 1–16. doi: 10.1007/s10586-017-0951-z.

Moreira, M. R. A., Gherman, M. & Sousa, P. S. A. (2017) Does innovation influence the performance of healthcare organizations? *Innovation: Management, Policy and Practice*, 19(3), 335–352. doi: 10.1080/14479338.2017.1293489.

National Health Service (2020) Ministry of Health, DGS. Available at: https://www.sns.gov.pt/institucional/ministerio-da-saude/ (Accessed on 14 April 2020).

National Health Service (2021) *Administração Central do Sistema de Saúde*. Available at: http://www.acss.min-saude.pt/?lang=en (Accessed on 16 March 2021).

OECD/Eurostat (2018) *Oslo Manual 2018, Handbook of Innovation Indicators and Measurement.* doi: 10.1787/9789264304604-en.

Pikkarainen, M., Hyrkäs, E. & Martin, M. (2020) Success factors of demand-driven open innovation as a policy instrument in the case of the healthcare industry. *Journal of Open Innovation: Technology, Market, and Complexity,* 6(2), 1–16. doi: 10.3390/JOITMC6020039.

Polónia, D. F. & Gradim, A. C. (2021) Innovation and knowledge flows in health-care ecosystems: The Portuguese case. *The Electronic Journal of Knowledge Management,* 18(3), 374–391. Available at: https://academic-publishing.org/index.php/ejkm/article/view/2122/1949 (Accessed on 7 April 2021).

Portugal 2020 (2020) *Centro 2020.* Available at: http://www.centro.portugal2020.pt/ (Accessed on 9 April 2020).

Russell, L. B. (1977) The diffusion of hospital technologies: Some econometric evidence. *The Journal of Human Resources,* 12(4), 482–502. doi: 10.2307/145371.

Sadeghifar, J., *et al.* (2014) The relationship between organizational learning and staff empowerment in hospital: A correlational study in Iran. *Asian Social Science,* 10(16), 27–33. doi: 10.5539/ass.v10n16p27.

Salge, T. O. & Vera, A. (2009) Hospital innovativeness and organizational performance: Evidence from english public acute care. *Health Care Management Review,* 34(1), 54–67. doi: 10.1097/01.HMR.0000342978.84307.80.

Schultz, C., Zippel-Schultz, B. & Salomo, S. (2012) Hospital innovation portfolios: Key determinants of size and innovativeness. *Health Care Management Review,* 37(2), 132–143. doi: 10.1097/HMR.0b013e31822aa41e.

Simões, J. (2009) Os sistemas de saúde nos países da OCDE nos últimos 25 anos. In: Almedina, E. (ed.) *Retrato político da saúde — Dependência do percurso e inovação em saúde: da ideologia ao desempenho,* 11th edn. pp. 29–72.

Smith, K. H. (2005) Measuring innovation. In: *The Oxford Handbook of Innovation.* Oxford University Press, New York, pp. 148–177.

Sorbie, A., *et al.* (2021) Examining the power of the social imaginary through competing narratives of data ownership in health research. *Journal of Law and the Biosciences,* 1–21. doi: 10.1093/jlb/lsaa068.

Suominen, A., Seppänen, M. & Dedehayir, O. (2019) A bibliometric review on innovation systems and ecosystems: A research agenda. *European Journal of Innovation Management,* 22(2), 335–360.

Tidd, J. (2021) A review and critical assessment of the ISO 56002 innovation management systems standard: Evidence and limitations. *International Journal of Innovation Management,* 24(1). doi: 10.1142/S1363919621500493.

van Veghel, D., Marteijn, M. & de Mol, B. (2016) First results of a national initiative to enable quality improvement of cardiovascular care by transparently reporting on patient-relevant outcomes. *European Journal of Cardio-thoracic Surgery*, 49(6), 1660–1669. doi: 10.1093/ejcts/ezw034.

Weng, R., *et al.* (2011) Determinants of technological innovation and its effect on hospital performance. *African Journal of Business Management*, 5(11), 4314–4327. doi: 10.5897/AJBM10.1339.

Weng, R. H., Huang, C. Y. & Lin, T. E. (2013) Exploring the cross-level impact of market orientation on nursing innovation in hospitals. *Health Care Management Review*, 38(2), 125–136. doi: 10.1097/HMR.0b013e31824b1c84.

Wu, I. L. & Hsieh, P. J. (2011) Understanding hospital innovation enabled customer-perceived quality of structure, process, and outcome care. *Total Quality Management and Business Excellence*, 22(2), 227–241. doi: 10.1080/14783363.2010.532343.

Yang, C. W. (2015) Implementing hospital innovation in Taiwan: The perspectives of institutional theory and social capital. *International Journal of Health Planning and Management*, 30(4), 403–425. doi: 10.1002/hpm.2248.

Yang, C. W., *et al.* (2017) The association of hospital governance with innovation in Taiwan. *International Journal of Health Planning and Management*, 33(1), 246–254. doi: 10.1002/hpm.2441.

Yang, Q., *et al.* (2020) Collaborated effort against SARS-CoV-2 outbreak in China. *Clinical and Translational Medicine*, 7–10. doi: 10.1002/ctm2.7.

Zweifel, P. (1995) Diffusion of hospital innovation in different institutional settings. *International Journal of the Economics of Business*, 465–482.

https://doi.org/10.1142/9781800614192_0003

Chapter 3

Building Innovation Management Support at a University Hospital

Ingrid Kihlander[†,‡,¶], Erika Bellander Nydahl[§], and Stefan Vlachos[*]

†*RISE Research Institutes of Sweden, Stockholm, Sweden*

‡*KTH Royal Institute of Technology, Stockholm, Sweden*

§*Karolinska University Hospital, Solna, Stockholm, Sweden*

¶*ingrid.kihlander@ri.se*

This chapter provides an illustration of how the support for innovation work has been developed at Karolinska University Hospital. Karolinska is a large university hospital in Sweden that provides highly specialised healthcare together with research and education. The chapter presents a 'journey' spanning the period 2011–2020 whose overall goal was to support innovation efforts at the hospital. During that time, different initiatives to achieve the goal were launched. These included establishing expertise in forming and leading innovation partnerships; developing a portfolio of educational programmes for clinical staff regarding innovation management; utilising the opportunity to certify the hospital's innovation management professionals; engaging in the development of ISO standards for innovation management; and designing and implementing a hospital-wide innovation management system. This journey is then reflected upon, and the specific issues of adapting innovation management to a healthcare context and developing innovation management support in a hospital setting are discussed. This all serves as input for how to address innovation management as well as for future models of healthcare delivery.

---

[*] Stefan Vlachos served as the Head of the Innovation Center at Karolinska University Hospital from 2015 to 2021.

1. Introduction

Karolinska University Hospital (Karolinska) is a large university hospital with a history of being a prominent care provider and promoter of research and innovation activities. This chapter focuses on how Karolinska actively worked to support innovation efforts and foster innovation capabilities.

An internal support function, the Center for Innovation (CfI) was established at the hospital in 2011. This chapter presents how Karolinska developed its approach for supporting innovation during 2011–2020, with CfI as an internal innovation hub. The main phases and key activities during this 10-year period are presented, and reflections on the following topics are discussed:

- Adaption and implementation of innovation management in the public sector related to an overall professionalisation in the field of innovation management that has its roots in the private sector.
- Aspects such as innovation management skills, roles and organisation related to supporting innovation efforts in a hospital.

With this as the point of departure, we contribute to the discussion by identifying implications for future models of healthcare delivery based on Karolinska's experiences and ambitions. We include literature on innovation in the studied context as well as the current stance on professionalisation within innovation management. We also present the case organisation, its context and how the study was conducted. Key phases and events in the development of the innovation support are presented in chronological order. Finally, the experiences are discussed, and implications defined from a number of perspectives.

1.1. *Innovation in hospitals*

Given the overarching aim in healthcare to improve the health of the population and the patient experience as well as to reduce associated costs (Berwick, Nolan and Whittington, 2014), there is an openness to developing new delivery models for the future. To address this, efforts aimed at enhancing innovation capabilities in hospital organisations have been identified as contributing to increasing clinical performance (Moreira, Gherman and Sousa, 2017; Salge and Vera, 2009), even if such results should, according to Dias and Escoval (2013), be interpreted with caution. Furthermore, although innovation initiatives in healthcare often have the stated aim of increased effectiveness and efficiency (De Vries, Bekkers and Tummers, 2016), providing clear evidence that these aims are met seems to pose a challenge (Moreira *et al.*, 2017; Salge and Vera, 2009).

Innovation may be challenging *per se*, but healthcare faces specific barriers that can be related to actor networks, complex systems for funding and remuneration, threats of litigation, territorial behaviour from potentially disrupted professionals, and barriers related to regulations and policy level (Gorman, 2015; Herzlinger, 2006).

In research on healthcare innovation, hospitals are usually investigated in their role as adopters of innovation (Salge and Vera, 2009); such research addresses diffusion, dissemination, implementation and adoption of innovation (Atun *et al.*, 2010; Greenhalgh *et al.*, 2004). Research on hospitals as generating, instead of adopting, innovation is rather limited. In addition, the available research on hospitals as innovators is quite heterogeneous and utilises a multitude of approaches and theoretical perspectives (Thune and Mina, 2016). This might, according to Djellal and Gallouj (2005), be related to an underestimation, or even non-recognition, of innovation efforts in hospitals. More research regarding innovation generated from within healthcare organisations has been sought (Salge and Vera, 2009). This chapter aims to tackle this request by sharing insights into internal hospital innovation efforts, as exemplified by Karolinska University Hospital. University hospitals can be considered important nodes for innovation in the healthcare system, connecting clinicians, academia and industry, shouldering a broad role that encompasses care, education and research (Thune and Mina, 2016), and enabling the linkage of diverse sources of knowledge that stimulate idea generation (Thune and Gulbrandsen, 2017).

Innovation activities in healthcare can use a more science-based mode for learning and innovation (science, technology and innovation mode) or a more practice-based mode (doing, using and interaction mode) (Salge and Vera, 2009). Science-based innovation can be seen as results from dedicated research and development conducted by specialist personnel, while practice-based innovation is motivated by issues encountered in everyday clinical practice and is often performed informally, involving different roles and hierarchical levels in the organisation. A bias to mostly science-based innovation work remains, though, among scholars and policymakers (Jensen *et al.*, 2007).

1.2. *Organising and managing innovation work*

Managing and organising innovation is complex and can involve challenges such as people's understanding of innovation; their attention spans and competencies; leadership and building innovation cultures; creating new value; and managing connections and part–whole relationships (Bessant, 2003; Van de Ven, 1986). Organisations have several choices regarding how to organise their innovation work. Bhattacharyya, Blumenthal and Schneider (2018) have identified a number of strategies for innovation in healthcare organisations with different cases illustrating either a closeness to senior leadership or a limited oversight from senior leadership, and either only specialised teams or high integration of clinical staff.

With care production as an omnipresent priority in healthcare organisations, bringing innovation into focus might pose a dilemma. Therefore, organisations can benefit from considering how they can be effective, both with a daily delivery focus as well as in exploring new opportunities, perhaps by separating tasks based on factors like organisational structure or timing (Tushman and O'Reilly III, 1996). Kötting and Kuckerz (2019), for example, recommend deploying a combination of exploration-oriented, exploitation-oriented and transformation-oriented (aiming to transform the corporate culture) programmes.

Having a dedicated innovation function can increase innovation activity in a healthcare organisation because it raises awareness of innovation in the organisation (Labitzke, Svoboda and Schultz, 2014). However, a dedicated innovation function might induce a more formal and centralised innovation process, potentially hampering creativity and drive and thus impacting innovation performance negatively (*ibid.*).

In idea generation and innovation, it is beneficial to use diverse knowledge sources, internal as well as external, and support interaction and co-production (Sehgal and Gupta, 2019; Thune and Gulbrandsen, 2017). Specifically, Paguet and Wald (2018) point out that professional organisations like hospitals should encourage more high-quality inter-actions among different professional roles, since a lack of connection between formal (more hierarchical) and informal (more relational) net-works can risk weakening the implementation of organisational innova-tions in daily practice. To actively support bridging this gap between different actors, knowledge brokering can be beneficial since it supports the utilisation and translation of knowledge from other fields that can be combined and applied in innovative ways in another domain (Hargadon, 2002). This is also applicable internally within the same organisation, where social structures can be mediated (Currie and White, 2012).

Interestingly, Bhattacharyya *et al.* (2018) point out that some of the most innovative healthcare organisations do not have a structure for inno-vation or specific training. Instead, they focus on creating possibilities for individuals and groups to explore opportunities while being backed by management. Salge and Vera (2009) emphasise the importance of creating a culture of 'organisational innovativeness', not limiting innovation man-agement to administrating a pipeline of innovation projects, through com-bining effective incentives and support functions. Hence, adopting a systemic and systematic approach to innovation management could be recommended (Karlsson and Magnusson, 2019).

1.3. *Professionalisation in innovation management*

An overall professionalisation can be identified in the field of innovation management. ISO, the International Organization for Standardization, is developing the standards family ISO 56000 including, e.g. ISO 56002:2019, Innovation Management System — Guidance, published in 2019. Research results from implementing innovation management sys-tems are still scarce, although positive effects related to increased capac-ity and results, and stronger promotion of all types of innovation, have been reported (Martinez-Costa, Jimenez-Jimenez and del Pilar Castro-del-Rosario, 2019; Mir, Casadesús and Petnji, 2016). Further, adoption of standardised innovation management in healthcare centres has been reported to result in consistent data collection, which contributes to better decision-making in the Spanish healthcare system (Moreno-Conde *et al.*, 2019).

Signs of professionalisation include the presence of specialisation, organisational structure, ways to ensure competence and skills levels (e.g. through certification) and a kind of exclusiveness (Evetts, 1999; Freidson, 1999). Within the field of innovation management, there is initial research that addresses what professional innovation leaders do (e.g. Maier and Brem, 2018). Personal certification related to innovation has been established fairly recently (e.g. Landry, 2016), and a personal certification for innovation management professionals complying with the standards ISO/ IEC 17024:2012, Conformity assessment — General requirements for bodies operating certification of persons (ISO, 2012) was developed in 2017 (Kihlander, Magnusson and Karlsson, 2022).

2. Methods and Materials

This section introduces the Swedish healthcare system, presents an in-depth case study at one hospital organisation, and describes how the study was conducted.

2.1. *Case and context*

2.1.1. *Healthcare in Sweden*

The Swedish healthcare system is almost entirely funded through taxes and is governed by legislation through the Healthcare Act, complemented by topic-specific legislation. Along with the National Board of Health and Welfare's regulations, these laws govern healthcare practice nationwide.

Sweden's 21 regions are responsible for organising the provision of healthcare so that it meets legal requirements and provides adequate access for its citizens. To do this, the regions collect taxes. The regions are thus the payers of healthcare and, in many cases, also the providers. However, many private providers also operate, particularly in primary care. The paying arm of the region sets up contracts with both the public care providers and the private care providers. These contracts typically specify the quantity of care, the type of care the region 'ordered' from the providers and how this care is remunerated, for example, based on DRG points (diagnosis-related group, a system for classifying hospital cases).

The 290 municipalities in Sweden are responsible for elderly care, rehabilitation care and other services required after discharge from the healthcare providers. For this, the municipalities also collect taxes. These services also typically have both public and private providers.

Lastly, there are private providers and a growing number of private insurances offered, outside the tax-funded system. The focus of this chapter, however, is on a public healthcare organisation.

2.1.2. *Karolinska University Hospital*

Sweden's Karolinska University Hospital (Karolinska) is one of the largest university hospitals in Europe. Karolinska has over 15,000 employees, 2,600 active researchers, 1,100 beds and 1.4 million patient visits per year. It has received recognition in global comparisons — *Newsweek*, for example, ranks it number 6 in the world based on recommendations from medical professionals, results from patient surveys and key medical performance indicators (*Newsweek*, 2023).

Region Stockholm is responsible for all publicly financed healthcare in the county of Stockholm. Karolinska is tasked with *providing highly specialised healthcare together with research and educating the professionals of tomorrow*. Further, Region Stockholm has defined an innovation strategy stipulating that all units are responsible for pursuing systematic innovation.

The hospital has recently undergone an extensive reorganisation in which a new operational model has been implemented. The clinical practice is now organised into six themes and three functions. The themes are specific to a theme of diagnoses, such as Cancer or Emergency & Reparative Medicine. The functions provide services across the themes and include Medical Diagnostics (imaging and lab) and Perioperative Medicine & Intensive Care.

CfI is a support function at Karolinska that serves as a competence centre for innovation, coaching the organisation with the goal to nurture internal innovation capabilities. CfI strategically works with innovations and partnerships in order to shape the best possible healthcare for the patients of tomorrow (Karolinska, 2021). Over the years the number of employees has shifted, from slightly over 10 people to over 20 people. CfI's evolution since its inception in 2011 is one of the strands of interest in this chapter.

2.2. *Research approach and methods*

Our study of one organisation, Karolinska, draws on case study methodology beneficial to capture a real-world case and its context (Eisenhardt, 1989; Yin, 2009). Further, the work has been carried out in collaboration between CfI practitioners and an innovation management researcher. This insider–outsider constellation leveraged the benefits of insider know-how, a contextual understanding and access to the organisation combined with the outsider's research perspective.

The empirical data were gathered in archival search and interviews. The archival search encompassed different types of reports (performed by both practitioners and researchers) and communication material, such as annual reports, presentation material and research reports. In addition, the practitioners also sought validation for the course of events in their personal archives of materials and notes, such as internal interviews related to CfI operations, calendars and written personal communications.

Interviews were conducted with the following three types of respondents for three different purposes. All interviews were conducted by the researcher, digitally recorded and transcribed.

• Key personnel at CfI: head of CfI, the person responsible for implementation of the Karolinska innovation management system, and CfI communications manager. The interviews aimed to capture history and current developments. Three respondents, nine interviews in total.
• Clinical personnel involved in innovation efforts supported by CfI. The interviews aimed to capture innovation work and how it was supported by CfI. Three respondents, one interview each.
• Certified innovation managers at CfI. Interviewed in order to reflect on their certification as innovation management professionals. Nine

people interviewed, one interview each, of which two also interviewed as key personnel.

The empirical data were compiled, reduced and arranged into a chronological description that identified key phases and events. These constitute the foundational structure in the next section, and as a subsequent step, the description was analysed based on the purpose defined at the study's outset.

3. Key Phases in Building Innovation Management Support

To describe the development from 2011 to 2020, four key phases were identified: Initiation of the CfI; Innovation partnerships with industry; Increasing innovation capability at the hospital and professionalising innovation management; and Holistic approach to support innovation. These four key phases, including a number of key events, are presented in chronological order. Reflections over actions taken and their perceived effects are also presented. An overview of the four phases is given in Figure 1.

3.1. *Phase 1: Initiation of the Center for Innovation*

CfI was established in 2011 with the ambition of bringing together healthcare, academia and industry to create patient value based on unmet healthcare needs, through joint innovation. The vision was to create an arena for interactions and for identification, training and further development of innovation methods and tools. This vision was reflected in the choice of name in Swedish for the centre, Innovationsplatsen, which literally means 'the place for innovation'. Different perspectives and competencies were brought together at CfI — nurses, doctors, bioengineers, IT/telecom consultants, a lawyer and experts on human–computer interaction, telemedicine and user-centred design, data science, communication, funding and business development.

The innovation initiatives supported by CfI were performed with a clear goal: more efficient care at a lower cost and more rapid

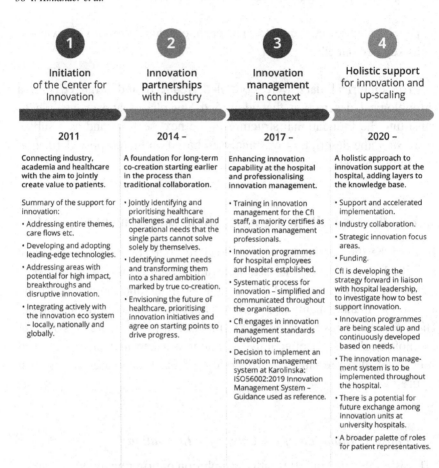

Figure 1.   Key phases in building innovation management support at Karolinska.

development of tomorrow's healthcare solutions. The initiatives aimed to achieve patient benefit as soon as possible and, simply put, to create maximum patient value for Swedish taxpayers' money. Therefore, CfI had no intention to commercialise employees' ideas or focus on technology transfer. Commercialisation services were, though, offered by other parties in the surrounding ecosystem, primarily the medical university connected to the hospital, Karolinska Institutet. Instead, the goal was to drive development by identifying new areas of innovation and to support innovation projects through to implementation in everyday clinical practice. The focus has, from the start, been broad, ranging from apps to entire care chains and work methods that encompass the development of new equipment and adoption of emerging technologies. Some of the earliest projects included taking cell therapy from the lab to the patient, as well as optimising the care pathway for patients who experience strokes or heart failure. Other initiatives focused on mobile health and e-health, analytics, radiotherapy, automation in the care sector, and patient influence in palliative care.

From the very start, medical professionals were seen as key resources in the development efforts. However, additional perspectives were also requested in order to cope with the major healthcare challenges. Therefore, Karolinska aimed to establish national and international partnerships among industry, academia and healthcare.

Though 'triple-helix constellations' (industry, academia, healthcare) was a buzzword at the time, industry partnerships had been a part of the hospital's development for years. The real novelty was to address the lack of structure in how to establish and drive such partnerships, a lack identified not only by Karolinska staff and leadership but also by representatives from the MedTech industry.

Processes were established that demonstrated step-by-step how to set up and drive these partnerships and provided guidance on managing expectations around joint innovation and how to proceed. A new collaboration model between healthcare and industry, Innovation Partnership, was developed with the goal to jointly transform healthcare, not only to collaborate around individual projects: *Together, we will change the organisation, processes and working methods of healthcare. Not only will we generate greater patient value, but also discover and create new forms of value.* The partnership model could be seen as an invention in itself.

At this time, CfI was part of a major central hospital resource for staff, Development and Innovation, that aimed to strengthen the developmental potential by gathering Medical Technology, IT, eHealth, cross-border care and CfI together. When a new state-of-the-art facility initially called

New Karolinska in Solna was scheduled to be built, yet another task was given to the staff: equip the new hospital building with medical technology.

Summary of support for innovation, Phase 1:
- Addressing entire themes, care flows and functional areas
- Developing and adopting leading-edge technologies
- Addressing areas with potential for high impact, breakthroughs and disruptive innovation
- Partnerships with industry, leading academic institutions and other world-leading hospitals
- Integrating actively with the innovation eco-system — locally, nationally and globally

---

3.2. Phase 2: Innovation partnerships with industry — a foundation for long-term co-creation

The second phase, starting in 2014, was characterised by the structured industry partnerships initiated in a competitive public procurement process.

Because of the major investment in life sciences in the Stockholm region and the construction of the new hospital building, Karolinska succeeded in taking the strategic industry partnerships to the next level (Permert, 2015). Investing billions of Swedish crowns opened a window of opportunity for healthcare to take the lead. In order to maximise the impact of taxpayer money, innovation partnerships were forged with companies that supplied equipment to the new hospital building. Not only should suppliers deliver up-to-date equipment over time, but they should serve as an attractive innovation partner.

The innovation partnerships linked to the procurement of MedTech equipment were initially established in 2014. Up to 14-year contracts were signed, with an extension option of six years. The commitments paved the way for long-term collaboration, where the development of a more systematic approach to both innovation efforts and collaboration models played a major part in building the CfI knowledge base. New partnerships have been added to the portfolio over time, and the scope has broadened from medical technology to encompass all kinds of procurement areas, such as patient meals.

When initiating an innovation partnership, focus areas for the joint innovation were selected to address unmet healthcare needs (e.g. connected care or minimally invasive surgery). Within each focus area, a variety of innovation projects was defined to address key healthcare challenges. Further, a well-tested process called the ABCD Model was used to systematically align the joint efforts within the innovation partnerships. The model encompasses four phases of joint innovation work: (A) Identification of unmet needs, (B) Scoping of project, (C) Execution of project, and (D) Translation into commercial and clinical implementation. The ABCD Model has been further developed and is a work in progress that adapts theory to practice and vice versa. Learnings from the first five years of the most active innovation partnership were consolidated in 2020 and used as input to a new strategic plan for influencing future collaboration. Based on in-depth needs analyses and workshops (including representatives from both organisations), the collective experience highlighted the importance of the following:

- Combining a formal governance process with informal relationships.
- Taking unmet needs, clinical and operational, as starting points for all innovation initiatives.
- Creating and enabling a structure for programme initiatives.

By addressing healthcare as a 'connected whole', the innovation partners can together unlock gains and efficiencies and drive innovation that help deliver on the quadruple aim: enhancing the patient experience, improving health outcomes, lowering the cost of care and improving the working life of care providers.

CfI has become Karolinska's knowledge hub for innovation collaboration with industry. Its mission is to continuously build knowledge on how to establish, drive and leverage innovation partnerships with industry — for the benefit of patients and hospital staff alike.

The Innovation Partnership developed in Phase 2 is a foundation for the following:
- Starting the discovery process early, to identify where industry and healthcare partners have common grounds and interests
- Jointly identifying and prioritising healthcare challenges and clinical and operational needs that the single parts cannot solve solely by themselves
- Identifying unmet needs and transforming them into a shared ambition marked by true co-creation
- Envisioning the future of healthcare, prioritising innovation initiatives and agreeing on starting points to drive progress

3.3. *Phase 3: Increasing innovation capability at the hospital and professionalising innovation management*

Phase 3, starting in 2017, was characterised by the ambition to develop innovation management in the context of a university hospital. The aim was to increase the ability to lead and spread innovation throughout the organisation, based on an increased use of evidence-based knowledge as well as practice-based innovation experience. Innovation skill sets, processes and tools, as well as how to lay the groundwork for taking a systems approach to innovation management, were addressed in this phase.

For CfI, internal innovation management training was an essential component. It provided a chance to strengthen knowledge of innovation management as well as establish a common framework for innovation management and for the role of an innovation management professional at the hospital. As a further demonstration of CfI's ambitious goals, a majority of the CfI staff began the process of becoming certified as innovation management professionals. Additionally, 'innovation manager' was defined as a formal role and became registered in the HR system.

Several training programmes that addressed innovation methods and strategy were launched for Karolinska employees and leaders: *Innovation Ambassador* — how to drive innovation projects, including design thinking methods; *Innovation for Leaders* — how to use innovation as a strategic tool and support innovative employees; and *Innovation Manager* — for employees with innovation management as a profession. In addition, a module on innovation strategy was also incorporated into the regular leadership programmes. Currently, more than 200 Karolinska employees have completed one of the innovation training programmes offered by CfI. The courses are in great demand, not only from within Karolinska but from other parts of the region and external actors. New educational concepts are continuously being created based on experiences and learnings. For example, a course targeting participants in innovation partnerships, gathering industry representatives and healthcare staff in the same classroom, was discussed. Furthermore, a first step towards a Healthcare Transformation Academy is being taken together with other European university hospitals, in which Karolinska's role is to continue developing innovation programmes tailored to the university hospital context.

Over time, CfI has developed the toolbox based on both empirical and theoretical knowledge in collaboration with clinical staff, innovation researchers and organisations aiming to professionalise innovation management. For example, related to the detailed step-by-step process developed in Phase 1, CfI has simplified the systematic innovation process in order to make it more accessible and easier to adapt. Further, in collaboration with researchers from health management and innovation management, how to best support innovation at the hospital was explored. It was identified that 'another manual' was not the silver bullet for efficiently supporting innovation efforts. Instead, CfI decided to offer a combination of personal coaching from experienced innovation managers and evidence-based theory to support the organisation.

Externally, development of the ISO standards was ongoing, and representatives from CfI got involved in the national innovation management standards committee. To make both the internal and external cumulative knowledge more tangible for the hospital employees and leadership, hospital management later decided to establish a hospital-wide support system, an innovation management system using guidance from ISO 56002:2019, based on CfI's recommendations. CfI was appointed as responsible for developing and implementing such a system at Karolinska. As an initial activity, CfI undertook a gap analysis that identified the current situation in the organisation as benchmarked against ISO 56002:2019. The analysis showed that many system elements could be identified as already present in the organisation, such as processes for service design and for external collaboration, but the real benefit was to use the system model presented in the standard. The system model provided a terminology and a logical structure for connecting the system elements. Taking a systems perspective is expected to bring benefits on a system level, not only from separate projects.

Phase 3 was characterised by an increased ambition to enhance innovation capabilities at the hospital, and to professionalise innovation management:
- Training in innovation management for entire CfI staff
- A majority of CfI staff gets certified as Innovation Management Professionals
- Innovation programmes for hospital employees and leaders established: Coaching programs for clinical staff (design thinking) and leadership programs: Innovation for leaders (innovation strategy)
- Systematic process for innovation — simplified and communicated throughout the organisation
- CfI engages in innovation management standards development
- Decision to implement an innovation management system at Karolinska: ISO 56002:2019 Innovation Management System — Guidance used as reference

3.4. *Phase 4: A holistic approach to supporting innovation*

Phase 4, starting in 2020, presents the CfI of today and its efforts to create a new strategy for best supporting innovation at the hospital, using a holistic approach and in close cooperation with hospital leadership and clinical departments.

CfI is now part of a central function that supports research, education, development and innovation capabilities at the hospital. Since a new step on the transformative journey is about to take place, CfI conducted a benchmark of innovation units at eight major European university hospitals during 2020. These units represented a variety in terms of maturity, size and mission. Some of them focused on innovation commercialisation, while others emphasised translational research. In the study, partnerships with industry and the ability to combine research and innovation were highlighted as challenging. Karolinska seemed to be the only hospital actively applying the ISO 56002 standard for innovation management systems at the time of the benchmark. Further, the Karolinska profile, with its strong emphasis on 'demand/needs-driven innovation', 'providing training', 'systematic innovation methodology' and 'industry collaboration', was found to be quite unique in this setting. The other participants expressed great interest in additional collaboration.

To shape the new strategy, in-depth interviews and dialogues with the directors were conducted to understand how they wanted to be supported by CfI — and which clinical needs most urgently required attention. This, alongside CfI's longstanding experience, analysis of future scenarios and opportunities brought on by emerging technologies and new knowledge, will help the hospital to point out next steps to take in order to increase capacity to support innovation efforts at the hospital.

With a dedicated CfI and the capabilities it builds up over time during different phases, Karolinska can forge systematic, long-term innovation initiatives. In concrete terms, this entails providing support for innovative healthcare solutions and enhancing the knowledge base among hospital staff, while improving prospects for future initiatives. Infrastructures are being improved so that healthcare can benefit from enabling technologies such as AI. CfI is also improving the ability to procure innovative resources and is thus enabling healthcare to be a driving force in innovation partnerships with industry. It is also important to allow people with patient experience and chronic conditions the latitude to become active participants in the developmental process, for example, in innovation project teams or by leading projects themselves.

CfI aspires to strengthen prospects for pursuing innovation based on the needs and challenges identified by the healthcare system that currently lack solutions. The overarching goal still remains — to create the best possible care for patients and healthcare personnel alike, today and tomorrow.

In a chronological presentation covering the year 2020, a reflection related to COVID is relevant. The pandemic has put intense pressure on several organisations, and hospitals in particular. Clinical staff as well as management are heavily burdened. However, the pandemic also highlighted some aspects to consider around systematic innovation. The pandemic functioned as a catalyst for scaling up innovation in response to the crisis and confirmed that a support function such as CfI plays an important role in paving the way for the future. In areas where CfI spent years developing new concepts (e.g. being proactive, performing analysis on needs and opportunities), some final barriers were suddenly removed enabling quick ramp-ups and implementation. For example, video visits increased 180% within a couple of weeks and cobots in the laboratory were quickly put to use. Innovation methods came in handy to handle new assignments and ramp up COVID testing capacity. The pandemic also created a sense of urgency around collaboration among care providers, for example, around innovation procurement — a need that became evident when the power balance shifted from procurer to supplier during the first stages of the pandemic and a lack of equipment emerged.

Phase 4 is characterised by the ambition to offer a holistic support for innovation and up-scaling, encompassing the following focus areas:

- Innovation support and accelerated implementation
- Industry collaboration
- Innovation focus areas
- Funding

CfI is developing the strategy forward in close cooperation with hospital leadership, including all directors, to investigate how to best support innovation.

- Innovation programmes are to be scaled up and continuously developed based on needs
- The innovation management system is to be further developed and implemented throughout the hospital
- Potential for future exchange among Innovation Units at European university hospitals
- A broader palette of roles is to be developed for patient representatives participating in innovation initiatives

4. Discussion of Identified Challenges and Experiences

The analysis of how to develop support for innovation efforts at the hospital from 2011 to 2020 provides several insights. We here share reflections on the identified challenges of adapting and implementing innovation management in a public sector setting, considering that much of innovation management professionalisation has its roots in the private sector regarding terminology and value models, for example. Further, we discuss the development related to previous research on innovation support and innovation management professionals.

4.1. *Major challenges identified when implementing innovation management in a public sector setting*

Over the years, Karolinska has experienced a number of major challenges to its innovation efforts and innovation management in the healthcare context. They resemble to a large extent what Herzlinger (2006) points out, such as regulatory barriers, complex actor networks and intricate financing and reimbursement systems. We elaborate on these challenges in the sections that follow.

4.1.1. *Goals and metrics for innovation in public services*

An overwhelming majority of literature and case studies on innovation, innovation management, entrepreneurship and intrapreneurship come from the private sector. Models, nomenclature and ultimate goals are formulated based on the premises that govern private enterprise, something that became evident in the internal training on innovation management arranged for CfI in Phase 3. This potential discrepancy was also identified as something that needed to be addressed in Karolinska's further work. Simply put, innovation goals in the private sector are often based around new products and services that have the potential to build and retain the customer base profitably. Whether profits are made by adding new product lines to existing operations or by spinning off growing units is secondary to shareholders, since they are just different ways of monetising successful innovation.

This approach is not, however, easily transferable to typical public services, which often face challenges formulating performance measurements (Dias and Escoval, 2013). Many public services exist not because more of them are desired *per se*, but because they are necessary in a civilised society. Social services are provided because people might need financial help or childcare during their life. Police authorities are needed to ensure safe communities, not because we want to see lots of people in uniform. Healthcare is provided because we sometimes get ill or hurt, not because we have an urge to be operated on a lot. Hence, many public services are available in order to help people when something unpleasant happens.

This means that growth, which is often generally identified as a motivator for innovation, is not a very good success metric for public services *per se*. Establishing proper innovation metrics for the public sector thus poses a challenge, since there is an inherent bias towards metrics rooted in a business context.

4.1.2. *Budgeting and legal limitations as boundary conditions*

Funding and co-creation with external parties are fundamental to innovation management, as Karolinska has demonstrated in its development of industry partnerships (formalised in Phase 2). However, public entities are subject to specific boundary conditions that differ from those of private sector companies. Specifically, revenues in a public organisation come from a budgeting process, not through sales, and collaboration with private companies is regulated through public procurement laws and state aid rules.

Public hospitals in Sweden operate on a yearly budget, and that budget mostly consists of payments for production according to a set framework often based on DRG points. Results are not carried over from one year to the next, so if the healthcare budget is not consumed within the budget year, there is a risk of receiving a reduced budget in subsequent years.

This is not necessarily a bad thing, since the point of many public services is not to grow and become bigger. However, the fact that the budget is reset every year makes it more challenging to run innovation initiatives that require several years to generate results. Behaviour is rather steered towards small improvements that can show an effect in a short period of time. Obviously, this favours highly incremental innovation and risks missing out on achieving more radical results. For example, for years Karolinska has put effort into testing and preparing for care visits via video, and deployed it to a somewhat limited extent. Yet, a broader scaling-up was not happening until the pandemic compelled it, even if the knowledge itself was developed earlier. However, without being able to perform the long-term work (in the absence of short-term benefits) this breakthrough would not have been possible.

Regulations for collaborating with private companies are primarily formulated according to the principle of equal and fair treatment of all companies. Thus, a public organisation must procure products and services through a public procurement process (with minor exceptions). Ultimately, the products or services that end up as part of daily operations (not part of clinical studies) must be procured this way.

Healthcare providers use lots of different technologies to provide their services, and much transformational innovation emerges from the combination of new technologies and new work approaches. These normally evolve and are developed in close collaboration among different companies and organisations as trial-and-error efforts, which show what works and what does not. So, finding a format for trial-and-error efforts *and* then implementing measures in daily operations is not at all straightforward for a public organisation. This was specifically addressed in the New Karolinska project, when collaboration was included as an add-on during procurement. Karolinska will continue to try and find ways to manage this.

4.1.3. *Value creation in healthcare — stakeholder value vs financial value*

Healthcare is complex. Several organisational entities are involved in providing care across a wide range of conditions, even more so when taking into account rehabilitation and the social security system.

Simply put, innovation in the private sector will move money from existing consumption to new consumption, sometimes at such a scale that the existing items consumed disappear while new items take over completely. The company that invests in producing a successful innovation is directly rewarded financially.

Financial flows in healthcare are not as direct. For example, the financial benefit almost always ends up in places other than where the innovation efforts originated. New procedures may well lessen the severity of disease by orders of magnitude by using new (and expensive) technologies and implementing new work approaches. For example, the case of optimising care pathways for heart failure patients (a task initiated in Phase 1) required a great effort in involving, persuading and co-developing with several affected units before the redesigned care path could be implemented. This also included some shifting of funds between departments. If successful, such results will be beneficial for the patients and also lower the costs of rehabilitation, social security or health insurance, for example, but will nevertheless probably result in higher costs for the treating clinical units.

4.2. *Developing innovation support for hospital-wide innovation capabilities*

The overarching goal — designing the best healthcare possible — has been the same ever since CfI was established, but the approach for achieving this has varied over time. Each step forward has been an explorative journey, with iterations and experiments just as any other innovation initiative. Insights have been gained gradually, and the CfI toolbox has evolved based on both empirical and theoretical knowledge in collaboration with several different actors. As CfI has learned and matured over time, the ambition levels have also progressed from being reactive to proactive and now to becoming systematic. Hence, a pattern of both a long-term ambition and an openness for testing and iterative learning surfaced in the analysis. This did not involve finding *the* final solution to supporting innovation in the hospital, but to pursuing continuous improvement of innovation support.

When summarising how the approach to innovation has developed at Karolinska during the specified time period, a number of perspectives identified in the analysis are interesting to further elaborate on. These include skills and roles related to innovation management in public healthcare, organising innovation support, the innovation management support's shift towards a systems approach and its implementation, and the necessity to keep the future in focus.

4.2.1. *Skills for innovation management in complex public healthcare settings*

In addition to the skills needed for innovation management, the experiences from Karolinska shed light on factors related to innovation in public organisations.

Although not formulated specifically in the early phases of CfI, it was obvious that different stakeholders had different aims that needed to be managed in order to successfully collaborate with industry and academia. The early phases focused on collaboration in specific projects and programmes, funded through external sources. Traditional project management skills were therefore sought, with some elements of human-centred design also applied in a few projects. The innovation process was described in line with a traditional stage-gated project process.

As CfI members gradually became involved in procurement for the new hospital building, the need for new skill sets emerged with regard to how to form innovation partnerships with the companies that won a number of the equipment procurement contracts. Therefore, skills related to the *public procurement process* were needed. This involves being able to motivate the choice of procurement method (there are various methods with different inherent degrees of freedom for further interaction) and to express desired results and effects, rather than the conventional way of simply stating strict requirements. Such skills also include evaluating proposed work methods and understanding how the respondents intended to staff their partnership organisations. This is important for being able to gauge whether you can build trust between the organisations. During the New Karolinska project, this know-how was largely provided by external sources but has been integrated in CfI's current skill set.

After the procurements for new facility were finalised, a new set of necessary skills became apparent: *building joint strategies* and framing them within the boundary conditions of the corresponding equipment contracts. In selecting focus areas, another skill became obvious: *expressing value* beyond financial outcome for the involved parties, since financial value is not the primary outcome for the supplier. Lastly, in each collaboration project, it is always important to be aware of whether a project must revert from the development phase to procurement. An even greater need to use the procurement tool proactively was identified at Karolinska, including an ability to challenge the market while still complying with public procurement laws and hence the ability to view the procurement process as a strategic enabler rather than a barrier to innovation.

Additionally, an innovation manager must, individually or in collaboration with other professionals, be able to *track monetary flows* among departments within their own organisation and between organisations and other agencies; this is closely related to the reflections made on value creation. This is essential in more transformative innovation efforts, as it may also change fundamental flows. Although a revised monetary flow is not unique to the public healthcare environment, the decision process for changing such a flow is very different. This is because a private-sector buyer 'simply' decides to spend money elsewhere, whereas public-sector decisions are ultimately political ones. On a tactical and strategic level, an accomplished innovation manager understands this, and will be able to proactively address this topic.

Phase 3 was characterised by a need to increase proactivity and thus professionalisation gradually increased. In any organisation, this means a need to increase or add more systematic approaches on all levels, strategic, tactical and operational. Further, since CfI serves a hospital approximately one thousand times larger than itself, it was necessary to train people throughout the organisation, and with that, the ability to both scale CfI's skill sets and to follow up and report on organisation-wide innovation efforts. Hence, this induced a shift from *doing* (projects) to *supporting* (the organisation). The professionalisation of innovation management was explicitly discussed within CfI. The certification of several CfI employees as innovation management professionals was aligned with the goal of becoming more professional as an innovation management expert group. In healthcare, which relies on evidence-based knowledge and domain expertise, the innovation management certification was perceived as contributing to a legitimisation of the post of innovation manager as a 'real job'.

Innovation managers at CfI can be considered knowledge brokers who support combining of knowledge from different domains and organisations, or different parts of the organisation (Currie and White, 2012; Hargadon, 2002). In its role as a public hospital that plays a central part in hospital–industry partnerships, innovation managers at Karolinska must be able to *make things happen in a network of people and external organisations* and successfully navigate this landscape. This can be intricate depending on both how and where the value is created, and on what Paguet and Wald (2018) identified as the challenges of gaps between formal hierarchical and informal relational networks. Finally, experiences from Karolinska emphasise a need for the innovation managers to demonstrate *persistence*, since innovation often involves a constant effort to address established structures, manage people averse to change and tackle current obstacles.

4.2.2. *Organising support for innovation*

Innovation support can be organised in several ways (Bhattacharyya *et al.*, 2018). Since its founding in 2011, CfI has aimed to boost the hospital's innovation capability. The visibility of CfI as a dedicated innovation function has probably helped to raise awareness of innovation in the organisation (Labitzke *et al.*, 2014). However, it can be reflected on that commitment from top management has shifted over the years. In Phase 4, the final phase, CfI believes that its efforts are fully anchored with the hospital's top management.

Due to the limited number of employees at CfI (about 10–15) that intend to support over 15,000 employees in the organisation, training all kinds of hospital employees is key. CfI has also decided to initiate alumni groups related to these training programmes. This, in turn, will build hospital-wide networks of people with a basic understanding of innovation, a goal partly inspired by the dual operating system defined by Kotter (2012).

Further, in the benchmark with European university hospitals, several differences were identified including size, funding and innovation management maturity. A continued knowledge exchange among the hospitals and a widened benchmark can offer interesting insights, since Karolinska cannot currently identify any other hospitals with a similar profile.

4.2.3.   *A systems approach to innovation management*

Support for innovation at Karolinska has gradually developed and can be said at present to utilise a systems approach. The innovation has always been a part of Karolinska as a university hospital, and its systems approach has grown stronger along the way, crystallising when it decided to implement an innovation management system. The systems approach entails addressing several system elements such as strategy, process, culture and performance collectively and recognising their interdependence (Karlsson and Magnusson, 2019). The healthcare context is characterised by risk minimisation and utilisation of validated knowledge, so using an ISO standard seems relevant for the creation of a management system for innovation.

The internal gap analysis that used the ISO standard for innovation management systems, ISO 56002:2019, revealed that many system elements already existed. The benefits of deploying the system description from ISO 56002:2019 were that it enabled the use of an innovation terminology and a structure for connecting the elements. This structure facilitates a systematic approach that addresses all elements in a holistic way while sometimes focusing on particular elements.

What is happening now at Karolinska can be called transformation-oriented efforts around innovation management (Kötting and Kuckerz, 2019). Identifying clear performance results that correspond to other early research results on implementing innovation management systems (Martinez-Costa *et al.*, 2019; Mir *et al.*, 2016) is somewhat challenging, since the performance measurements themselves are under development. However, patience combined with an innovation unit empowered to take a long-term focus is necessary when building organisational capabilities for innovation and renewal. This was acutely illustrated in the pandemic, when the long-term innovation efforts reaped the benefits and could be promptly implemented when needs escalated.

Gains from taking an explicitly stated systems approach to innovation (Karolinska communicates that 'we are systematically pursuing innovation', not merely 'implementing an innovation management system') include the many different forms of innovation built up and supported by the organisation. Different mechanisms, such as methods, structures, leadership and performance measurements, can all support innovation since there is also a broad range in how innovation activities are performed, covering both science-based and practice-based innovation efforts (Salge and Vera, 2009).

Several implementation activities are being run in parallel and are directed at different target groups (clinical units, management, external actors). For example, training has been identified as key in building innovation capabilities utilising a bottom-up approach, and new educational concepts are therefore continuously developed.

To sum up Karolinska's systematic systems approach to its innovation efforts, it is clear that it develops both operations and employees alike.

4.2.4. *Future in focus*

This chapter has presented experiences from the perspective of a support function for innovation and innovation management in a large hospital. Its main task is to pave the way for innovation and new value creation while meeting the challenges and future needs of healthcare. This certainly became evident during the COVID-19 pandemic, when the hospital and healthcare system were cast right into the centre of the crisis. As a result of CfI's previous measures (analysing future scenarios, supporting external collaboration, and supporting systematic development and testing of possible solutions), the hospital could respond to the crisis by deploying these tested measures from its systematic innovation efforts. The increase in video visits and higher automation in the laboratory triggered by the crisis serve as proof that previous efforts in systematic innovation paid off. In parallel, CfI's role was not to be in the centre of the ongoing COVID crisis but to continue focusing on the future in order to develop relevant capabilities for analysing and addressing future scenarios. Figure 2 illustrates how systematic innovation efforts contribute to successful crisis management.

5. Implications for Future Models of Healthcare Delivery

Based on the experiences from Karolinska, a number of implications for future models of healthcare delivery can be formulated. First, there is no *one* specific model that we recommend. This study rather points to the

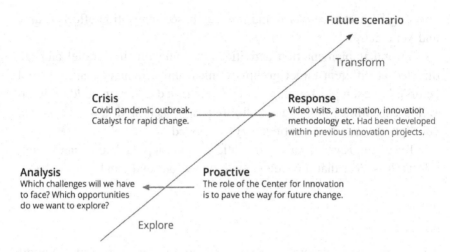

Figure 2.   How systematic innovation efforts at Karolinska contributed to the COVID-19 pandemic response.

importance of long-term ambitions for building support and an openness to exploring how innovation can be supported. Second, an innovation support function should never lose sight of the future, even during tough times.

In addition to these overall recommendations, the experiences of Karolinska captured in this study can serve as inspiration for hospitals as well as other healthcare system actors in shaping future models of healthcare delivery. Based on this study, areas that can be developed for innovation support are summarised in the following and are illustrated in Figure 3.

For organisations inspired by Karolinska's experiences, we can recommend taking a systems approach to managing innovation. Deploying an explicitly stated *systems approach for innovation management* enables support of the broad range of innovation activities in a complex hospital setting. Further recommendations include key measures like establishing an innovation *terminology* that really works in the specific context and finding ways to *combine top-down and bottom-up* approaches to achieve the desired impacts of systematic innovation efforts. In addition, we expect that a focus on *knowledge sharing* among hospitals, specifically

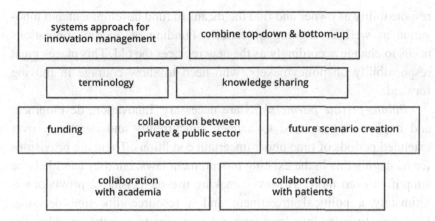

Figure 3.   Areas to include in developing innovation support for shaping future models of healthcare delivery.

among their innovation units, will be beneficial for the hospitals and for developing the field of innovation management in the university hospital context.

Implications for future models of healthcare delivery can also be identified as related to funding and collaboration that address practitioners (private and public organisations as well as patients), academia and policymakers, implying a fair amount of change. Healthcare is one of the most complex industries due to a mix of public and private providers, direct and indirect links among different parts of the social security system, and financial gains that are realised in other parts of the system than where the innovation investment takes place. Successful change in such complex systems needs to be emergent, meaning that it must consist of a fair amount of experimentation and trial and error. No singular organisation can accomplish this change on its own. This is exactly what innovation management is all about.

Funding for shaping transformative change in such a complex environment should be separated from funding of the daily operations, since current and future operational models will greatly differ. The new environment will replace the old, and this must happen through conscious decisions. In a setting where healthcare is both publicly funded and delivered, the public owner of the public healthcare provider needs to shoulder its responsibility as owner and find the means to fund development and innovation as well as ongoing operations. Funding of ongoing operations needs to change accordingly as the new replaces the old. This places great responsibility on policymakers, who need to show courage in moving forward.

Public–private partnerships are necessary. Innovation, development and implementation need to happen concurrently and iteratively over extended periods of time under uncertain conditions. There are provisions for managing this in the existing procurement laws, but they can likely be simplified even more. However, making use of legislative provisions is ultimately a political investment and a resource-allocation decision. Decisions to enter into long-term relationships to together develop the future represent a decision to invest under a high degree of uncertainty. This demands political courage.

To secure future relevance, *future scenarios* should be created. This requires skills in capturing and analysing the current and future needs, experiences and conditions of citizens, as well as describing the scenarios in a way decision-makers can understand. This will then enhance successful prioritising for present needs as well as proactive innovation efforts.

Collaboration with academia is also important. Again, in a highly complex world, there is no given linear progression from academic research through innovation to implementation and scaling. Academic research, as well as innovation and development, will all lead the way; for example, academic research can follow actual outcomes from continuous innovation efforts in a healthcare system.

Finally, *collaboration with patients* should not be forgotten. The patient, as a source of both needs and opportunities and a partner in collaboration, can increase the relevance of innovation efforts even further, contributing important perspectives.

5.1. *Future research*

For future research, the experiences of Karolinska point to several interesting strands. A strand of major interest would be how to build organisational capabilities that support both science-based and practice-based innovation, within the same organisation and how they can contribute to coping with the future that healthcare faces. This will require a systems approach when building the knowledge, since systems components such as organisation, structure, culture, leadership and performance must be studied and addressed in a holistic way.

References

Anderson, S., Nasr, L. & Rayburn, S. W. (2018) Transformative service research and service design: Synergistic effects in healthcare. *The Service Industries Journal*, 38(1–2), 99–113.

Atun, R., De Jongh, T., Secci, F., Ohiri, K. & Adeyi, O. (2010) Integration of targeted health interventions into health systems: A conceptual framework for analysis. *Health Policy and Planning*, 25(2), 104–111.

Bessant, J. (2003) Challenges in innovation management. In: Shavinina, L. V. (ed.) *International Handbook on Innovation*. Pergamon, pp. 761–774.

Berwick, D. M., Nolan, T. W. & Whittington J. (2008) The triple aim: Care, health, and cost. *Health Affairs*, 27(3), 759–769.

Bhattacharyya, O., Blumenthal, D. & Schneider, E. C. (2018) Small improvements versus care redesign: Can your organization juggle both? *NEJM Catalyst*, January.

Currie, G. & White, L. (2012) Inter-professional barriers and knowledge brokering in an organizational context: The case of healthcare. *Organization Studies*, 33(10), 1333–1361.

De Vries, H., Bekkers, V. & Tummers, L. (2016) Innovation in the public sector: A systematic review and future research agenda. *Public Administration*, 94(1), 146–166.

Dias, C. & Escoval, A. (2013) Improvement of hospital performance through innovation. *The Health Care Manager*, 32(2), 129–140.

Djellal, F. & Gallouj, F. (2005) Mapping innovation dynamics in hospitals. *Research Policy*, 34(6), 817–835.

Eisenhardt, K. M. (1989) Building theories from case study research. *The Academy of Management Review*, 14(49), 532–550.

Evetts, J. (1999) Introduction, Professions: Changes and continuities. *International Review of Sociology*, 9(1), 75–85.

Freidson, E. (1999) Theory of professionalism: Method and substance. *International Review of Sociology*, 9(1), 117–129.

Greenhalgh, T., Robert, G., Macfarlane, F., Bate, P. & Kyriakidou, O. (2004) Diffusion of Innovations in service organizations: Systematic review and recommendations. *The Milbank Quarterly*, 82(4), 581–629.

Gorman, D. (2015) On the barriers to significant innovation in and reform of healthcare. *Internal Medicine Journal*, 45(6), 597–599.

Hargadon, A. B. (2002) Brokering knowledge: Linking learning and innovation. *Research in Organizational Behavior*, 24, 41–85.

Herzlinger, R. E. (2006) Why innovation in health care is so hard. *Harvard Business Review*, 84(May), 58–66.

ISO, International Organization for Standardization (2012) ISO/IEC 17024:2012 *Conformity Assessment — General Requirements for Bodies Operating Certification of Persons.*

ISO, International Organization for Standardization (2019) ISO 56002:2019 *Innovation Management — Innovation Management System — Guidance.*

Jensen, M. B., Johnson, B., Lorenz, E. & Lundvall, B. Å. (2007) Forms of knowledge and modes of innovation. *Research Policy*, 36(5), 680–693.

Karlsson, M. & Magnusson, M. (2019) The systems approach to innovation management. In: Chen, J., Brem, A., Viardot, E. & Wong, P. K. (eds.) *The Routledge Companion to Innovation Management*. Routledge, pp. 72–90.

Karolinska (2021) Center for Innovation. Available at: https://www.karolinska hospital.com/research-innovation/innovation/ (Accessed on 1 February 2021).

Kihlander, I., Magnusson, M. & Karlsson, M. (2022) Certification of Innovation Management Professionals: Reasons for and Results from Acquiring Certification. *Journal of Innovation Management*, 10(1), 58–75.

Kotter, J. P. (2012) Accelerate: How the most innovative companies capitalize on today's rapid fire strategic challenges. *Harvard Business Review*, 90, 43–58.

Kötting, M. & Kuckertz, A. (2019) Three configurations of corporate innovation programs and their interplay. *European Journal of Innovation Management*, 23(1), 90–113.

Labitzke, G., Svoboda, S. & Schultz, C. (2014) The role of dedicated innovation functions for innovation process control and performance — An empirical study among hospitals. *Creativity and Innovation Management*, 23(3), 235–251.

Landry, D. (2016) The case for certification of the innovation professional. *International Journal of Innovation Science*, 8(1), 27–38.

Maier, M. A. & Brem, A. (2018) What innovation managers really do: A multiple-case investigation into the informal role profiles of innovation managers. *Review of Managerial Science*, 12, 1055–1080.

Martinez-Costa, M., Jimenez-Jimenez, D. & del Pilar Castro-del-Rosario, Y. (2019) The performance implications of the UNE 166.000 standardised innovation management system. *European Journal of Innovation Management*, 22(2), 281301.

Mir, M., Casadesús, M. & Petnji, L. H. (2016) The impact of standardized innovation management systems on innovation capability and business performance: An empirical study. *Journal of Engineering and Technology Management*, 41(July–September), 26–44.

Moreira, M. R. A., Gherman, M. & Sousa, P. S. A. (2017) Does innovation influence the performance of healthcare organizations? *Innovation*, 19(3), 335–352.

Moreno-Conde, A., Parra-Calderón, C. L., Sánchez-Seda, S., Escobar-Rodríguez, G. A., López-Otero, M., Cussó, L., del-Cerro-García, R., Segura-Sánchez, M., Herrero-Urigüen, L., Martí-Ras, N., Albertí-Ibarz, M. & Desco, M. (2019) ITEMAS ontology for healthcare technology innovation. *Health Research Policy and Systems*, 17(47).

Newsweek (2023) *The World's Best Hospitals 2023*. Available at: https://www. newsweek.com/rankings/worlds-best-hospitals-2023 (Accessed August 2023).

Pauget, B. & Wald, A. (2018) Creating and implementing organizational innovation: The role of professional identity and network embeddedness in healthcare organizations. *European Journal of Innovation Management*, 21(3), 384–401.

Permert, J. (2015) Innovation partnerships shaping the future of healthcare. Life Science in Sweden. Available at: https://www.karolinska.se/contentassets/ 95f7bf9087404aadaf8383f50eef0d77/innovationpartnership_byjohanper mert.pdf (Accessed on 1 March 2021).

Salge, T. O. & Vera, A. (2009) Hospital innovativeness and organizational performance: Evidence from English public acute care. *Health Care Management Review*, 34(1), 54–67.

Sehgal, S. & Gupta, G. (2019) Converging resources and co-producing for innovation: Evidence from healthcare services. *European Journal of Innovation Management*, 23(3), 429–453.

Thune, T. & Mina, A. (2016) Hospitals as innovators in the health-care system: A literature review and research agenda. *Research Policy*, 45(8), 1545–1557.

Thune, T. M. & Gulbrandsen, M. (2017) Combining knowledge to generate novelty: A study of disclosed ideas for life science inventions. *European Journal of Innovation Management*, 20(3), 446–462.

Tushman, M. L. & O'Reilly III, C. A. (1996) Ambidextrous organizations: Managing evolutionary and revolutionary change. *California Management Review*, 38(4), 8–29.

Van de Ven, A. (1986) Central problems in the management of innovation. *Management Science*, 32(5), 590–607.

Yin, R. K. (2009) *Case Study Research: Design and Methods* (4th edn.). Sage.

https://doi.org/10.1142/9781800614192_0004

Chapter 4

VIENNO — Vienna Innovation Model — Hacks the Healthcare

Mozghan Sadr[*,‡] **and Peter Granig**[†,§]

VAMED KMB, Vienna, Austria

†*University of Applied Science, Villach, Austria*

‡*mozhgan.sadr@vamed.com*
§*p.granig@fh-kaernten.at*

Hackathons are events that are based on the concept of open innovation, where organisations open up their innovation processes to internal and external participants to develop new ideas and solutions. Due to the wide range of applicability, hackathons have been used across industries to foster innovation and problem solving. However, several factors have to be considered regarding the organisation of these events, which need further improvements for better outcomes. At this point, the Vienna Innovation Model (VIENNO), which makes organisations aware of the inclusion of the ecosystem and its holistic view, can be used as a framework to organise efficient and innovative hackathons with greater success. VIENNO allows large, established healthcare organisations to imagine the future of healthcare. By eliminating some of the perceived risks, hackathons can be an effective way for large organisations to deliver breakthrough innovations at start-up speed. VIENNO hacks the old processes focusing on a concrete output in its cross-functional structure by fostering a patient-centric and can-do culture.

1. Introduction

In recent years, the ideation process has changed significantly in organisations. Due to the increasing number of competitors and growing dynamic markets, companies have to find new ways to create and develop innovative ideas. A well-known method is open innovation, which means that the doors of an organisation are opened, and ideas or needs of external individuals and other institutions are included in the product or service development. One application of this concept is the hackathon, a collaborative and competitive event where participants generate creative ideas within a very short time. These ideas can then be produced or developed in subsequent steps. These events bring participants from different backgrounds and professions together and enable them to work and collaborate in teams to address concrete problems and create prototypes by using the resources at their disposal. While hackathons were once reserved for software development, they have increasingly shifted into the mainstream in recent years and are now carried out in nearly all industries (Briscoe, 2014).

The innovation model VIENNO, developed by the Vienna General Hospital, VAMED-KMB and the Carinthia University of Applied Sciences, represents a collaborative approach that has been thoroughly tested and implemented in one of the world's largest hospitals. VIENNO represents the most adaptive and co-creative holistic innovation management model. This model aims to strengthen the capacity of organisations, communities, institutions and systems to respond to the growing drive of disruptive challenges through an innovation ecosystem that activates the major players. This model creates an ecosystem awareness that encourages decision-makers to participate in a joint journey from seeing only their own viewpoint (ego awareness) to experiencing the system from a common perspective while considering the whole system (eco awareness). The three pillars of the ecosystem are governments, corporations and society, which are represented in VIENNO and act equally in generative innovation development. In this way, VIENNO produces purposeful and future need-based innovations through co-sensing, co-inspiring and co-creation (Sadr and Granig, 2019). This model lays a foundation for sound and promising hackathons, especially in healthcare, its home sector.

As the hackathons are spread progressively into the mainstream, we have decided to take a close look at those that have been conducted in the last five years. Our study aims to (1) identify industries that already use this new form of open innovation while focusing on healthcare and (2) find out which hackathons have been successful and which ones have not, and why. Based on these objectives, this chapter compares VIENNO with the studied hackathons and underlines the advantages of this newly developed model.

2. Research Design

The present work demonstrates an unsystematic narrative review of the literature in which current scientific articles are summarised in a compact form (Green, Johnson and Adams, 2006). For this purpose, we searched for existing research results and articles on performing hackathons in different industries.

Research began in January 2020 by collecting basic information on the planning and implementation of hackathons to gain an overview of the topic and be able to assess the state of research. The databases PubMed, Medline and EBSCO were used. Google Scholar was also used but only for full-text search and source checking. To narrow the topic, we have defined the inclusion and exclusion criteria as follows.

Only studies and articles conducted between 2015 and 2019 (not older than five years) were included. Since hackathons have become more important across industries in recent years and have been performed increasingly, this study only included hackathons that were scientifically supported.

3. Research Results

In this chapter, the selected articles are presented in Table 1. We found a total of 27 articles concerning 9 different industries; these articles met the inclusion criteria and provided enough information on positive and negative aspects of the organisation. This was followed by an industry-specific classification. In addition, the lessons learned are highlighted for each hackathon.

Table 1. Hackathons held between 2015 and 2019 in industries supported scientifically.

Name	Industry	Date	Venue	Topic/Background	Participants	Lessons learned	Source
Farming							
Agriculture Data Hackathons	Agriculture	2016–2018	Netherlands	Data visualisation for pie farmers Drones, satellites and crop protection From farmer to city Network technology and sustainable livestock farming Manure hack Smart dairy farming Fishing hack Soil hack achterhoek Tractor hack National Soil Hack	6–22 local citizens	A correlation exists between participants' motivation and the distributed roles within the teams → integrating different strategies into the organisation of hackathons, which are tailored to all types of participants (e.g. citizens need to be involved differently from developers or problem owners)	Purwanto et al. (2019)
Culture							
Open Cultural Data Hackathon Coding Da Vinci — Bring the Digital Commons to Life	Culture	2016	Hamburg	Opening the digital data of Hamburg State and University Library to the public Use of digital data outside the cultural institutions	100 participants: software developers, designers, scholars and specialists from 19 cultural institutions in Northern Germany, Denmark and Sweden, working in 17 teams	Hackathon contributed to cultural awareness	Theise (2017)

Education

Consulting Hackathon	Education	2018	School of Entrepreneurship Israel	Innovation strategy Innovating branding and marketing strategy Optimising the company's sales processes	A total of 60 participants: 22 students, 22 company representatives, 16 mentors and experts	Importance of informing participants about the topic prior to the event In a one-day event, the teams should be smaller (with four members) Duration of event: one day is too short	Maaravi (2018)

Research

Evidence Synthesis Hackathon	Research	2018	Not mentioned	Solving some of the major issues facing evidence synthesis when using technology	25 programmers from across the world	Non-competitive nature of the event evaluated positively More focused topics, more qualified outcomes Pursuing sponsorship for hackathon	Haddaway and Westgate (2018)

Media

Nordisk Panorama Hackathon	Media Industries	2017	Denmark	Part of the Nordisk Panorama (NP) Film Festival Hackathon format to facilitate cross-disciplinary learning and innovation for filmmakers, developers and designers	26 participants (16 male, 10 female) 7 groups Some participants were selected by application and others were invited by the organisers	The perception of the participants based on their knowledge about hackathons was that programming skills are required and they were worried about not being able to contribute effectively	Karlsen and Løvlie (2017)

(Continued)

Table 1. (*Continued*)

Name	Industry	Date	Venue	Topic/Background	Participants	Lessons learned	Source
				Duration: 48 h		The authority of some participants was perceived as a hurdle for effective contribution of others. Using suitable facilitation tools can encourage the participants and improve the performance	Giffard-Roisin et al. (2018)
Meteorology							
The 2018 Climate Informatics Hackathon: Hurricane Intensity Forecast	Environment	2018	Colorado, USA	Prediction of the intensity of tropical and extra-tropical storms (24-h forecast) using information from past storms since 1979	38 participants (including 18 students) Expertise: 40% climate/weather 70% computer science 12 teams of 3 to 4 people	The participants had the opportunity to revise or rethink ideas and codes developed during the hackathon, after the hackathon was assessed positively	

Urban Development

World Heritage Meets Smart City in an Urban-Educational Hackathon in Rauma	Culture/Cities/Education	2018	Rauma Finland	Integration of historical uniqueness with modern city services in the City of Rauma with a World Heritage Old Town Combined educational–urban hackathon Smart cities	Students from one Research, Development and Innovation (RDI) class at Helsinki International Schools (HEI), majoring in technical or business subjects Organised by two HEIs and the Entrepreneur Association of Rauma	Dual focus is possible (should be included in the planning process) Involvement of universities and students in the innovation process of cities proved to be positive The public may be invited to have access to a more diverse set of expertise among the participants	Suominen *et al.* (2019)
Urban Hackathon	Cities/Urban Development	2015	Maribor	Renewal of the old city centre of Maribor Three two-day events in January ("City Toolbox: Revive the City Together"), April ("Reviving Koroška street") and October ("Reviving the city centre")	40–60 participants/event Municipal officials, university researchers (architect and traffic engineers), experts from different fields of urban development, representatives of NGOs, civil	Broad stakeholders' participation proved to be positive Largely contributed to improved access to information and problem solving Good approach to activate citizens and change their role	Pogačar and Žižek (2016)

(Continued)

Table 1. (*Continued*)

Name	Industry	Date	Venue	Topic/Background	Participants	Lessons learned	Source
				The hackathon resulted from the municipalities' inability to solve problems of economic, physical and social degradation	initiatives, students and local citizens	from passive consumers to active participants	
Technology and Big Data							
Think Tank Hackathon	Big Data	2018	Ljubljana	Follow-up of the "Big Data Training School for Life Sciences" held in Sweden Handling big data in life sciences Exchange of substantial knowledge about leading technologies Two-day event	8 participants Only open to attendees of the original training school in Sweden	Organising social activities for the participants prior to the event helps them get to know each other better, and promotes their cooperation during the event Suggesting improvements is easier than applying them in practice	Schulze *et al.* (2018)

Hack the Brain Hackathons	Technology and Health	2016	Amsterdam and Prague (2 hackathons)	Engaging the international artistic community to experiment with brain–computer–interface technologies and work with the scientific community to form an emerging neuro–art community	Engineers, programmers, designers	Importance of supporting the teams by mentors during the whole event (e.g. in ideation process) · Provision of information prior to the event raises the productivity of teams (online platforms can be used for this purpose) · Team-building activities support collaboration and spark the development of innovative ideas · Need to improve the evaluation and documentation tools	Valjamae *et al.* (2017)
Lab Hackathon (Pilot Hackathon)	Technology	2018	Zimbabwe, Africa	Building frugal and reproducible pieces of laboratory equipment to react to laboratory equipment shortages in Africa	Computer science, mechanical/electrical engineering, life/ natural sciences, economics, marketing and other social sciences · 13 teams registered, with an average of 6 members per team	Some issues revolved around the transfer of funds from the UK · Importance of providing support and information for participants	Webb *et al.* (2019)

(Continued)

Table 1. (*Continued*)

Name	Industry	Date	Venue	Topic/Background	Participants	Lessons learned	Source
Microsoft's One Week Hackathon	Technology	2017	Redmond	Four-day hackathon Largest hackathon organised by Microsoft For employees to develop ideas and projects they are mainly interested in	6,700 participants 1,800 projects	Motivation and project management are important success factors Involving future stakeholders supports the continuation of the started process Skill matching: tasks within teams should be distributed with regard to the individual skill levels rather than their own interest	Nolte *et al.* (2018)
Big Data Hackathon	Big Data	2016	Lyngby–Taarbæk	Smart city initiative in Lyngby–Taarbæk municipality	65 participants, mainly university students	Helpfulness of communicating predefined questions and problems for a better orientation	Jetzek (2015)

				Applied the triple helix model to create an informal collaboration between academia, government and private industry. Developing smart city solutions 48-h		Importance of team building and networking. Motivating the participants by a cash prize and giving students an opportunity to present their ideas to prominent industry members	
The CATS Hackathon by Cybersecurity Assessment Tools Project	Technology	2018	Not mentioned	For two days. To create and improve existing draft multiple-choice test items for a Cybersecurity Concept Inventory and Cybersecurity Curriculum Assessment	Cybersecurity educators and professionals from government and industry. 17 participants were organised into several teams, each with three or four members	Size of teams, duration of event and structure of event worked well. Diversity of the participants and interactions among them contributed greatly to the event's success. A challenge was finding experts who were willing to devote their time	Sherman *et al.* (2019)

(Continued)

Table 1.   (*Continued*)

Name	Industry	Date	Venue	Topic/Background	Participants	Lessons learned	Source
Soundscape Hackathon	Urban Planning and Design	2019	Ghent, Belgium	48 h To redesign and improve the soundscape of urban open spaces using virtual reality visualisation and ruralisation technologies	14 participants; local citizens and experts in 4 teams	Increasing diversity among participants would lead to more creativity Participants indicated that multiple smaller awards for different sub-challenges, instead of one team winning everything — could stimulate collaboration Scheduling enough time for final presentation is important	De Winne et al. (1932)
INSPIRE Hackathons	Environment–Big Data	Since 2014	INSPIRE Conference	Environmental information To combine open data, volunteered geographical information, GNSS and data from citizens observatories or other citizen science activities To use existing projects of the EU for further development	Developers, researchers, designers and others interested in open data, volunteered geographic information and citizen observatories	Building and maintaining networks help to exchange knowledge and expertise and train younger talents	Charvat et al. (2018)

Healthcare

MIT Hacking Medicine	Healthcare	2016	11 countries 9 US States Over 80 hackathons during the last 5 years	Student-, academic- and community-led innovation group that uses systems-oriented "healthcare hacking" to address the challenges in innovation adoption To develop new medical devices, digital health tools and solutions improving patient experience	500+ participants in each event Participants were all part of the healthcare ecosystem: engineers, scientists, clinicians, entrepreneurs and designers	MIT Hacking Medicine managed to help launch nearly 20 active companies that have raised over $120 M in financing. For this success, they received the 2016 Stanford Medicine X Healthcare Design Award, in the category of Education in Healthcare MIT Hacking Medicine model enables organisers to involve local stakeholders and experts	Lee (2016)
CAMTech Healthcare Hackathons	Healthcare	2012–2015	India Uganda USA	Focus on medical technology innovation to improve healthcare in resource-constrained settings	Number of participants is not mentioned: 12 hackathons (3 of them in cooperation with MIT Hacking Medicine)	CAMTech health hackathon model can drive the development of promising innovations	Olson *et al.* (2017)

(Continued)

Table 1. (*Continued*)

Name	Industry	Date	Venue	Topic/Background	Participants	Lessons learned	Source
				The Consortium for Affordable Medical Technologies (CAMTech) has developed a three-pronged model to maximise the effectiveness of hackathons: 1. Preceding priming activities focus on subsequent work 2. 48-h hackathons catalyse innovations 3. A suite of post-hackathon offerings stimulates the progress of innovations towards commercialisation	48-h operating phase	Driving factors of success: fundraising, prototyping, patenting, trailing, company formation, licensing and supporting structures for post-hackathon phase	
Mount Sinai Health Hackathon	Healthcare	2017	California	To harness the power of multidisciplinary and transdisciplinary collaboration and foster innovation in oncology using technologies using a format adapted from	87 participants representing 17 organisations; backgrounds in bioinformatics, software and hardware, product design, business,	No detailed information is available	Gabrilove *et al.* (2018)

| Health++ | Healthcare | 2016 | Stanford University | To collaborate, brainstorm and build solutions for unmet clinical needs Using a format adapted from guidelines provided by MIT Hacking Medicine 48 h | digital health and clinical practice 257 participants in interdisciplinary teams of students and professionals | Important considerations Limiting the team size to a maximum of six Considering gender and expertise balance Having well-defined evaluation criteria Business expertise is as critical as medical expertise Pre-hackathon: teaching a common framework of knowledge for medical innovation | Wang et al. (2018) |

(Continued)

Table 1. (*Continued*)

Name	Industry	Date	Venue	Topic/Background	Participants	Lessons learned	Source
						Post-hackathon: the development of ideas should be promoted even 3–6 months after the hackathon. Examples of fostering motivation and participation are monetary prices and investor networking opportunities	
Hackathon Hosted by Washington State University	Healthcare	2018	Washington	To solve rural health problems in Washington	Not mentioned	It may be helpful to include librarians with expertise in health sciences and business. This can attract support from the participants because librarians can take over research and library services, and enable participants to spend more time on prototyping Organisers and experts should have frequent and regular contact with the teams	Shin *et al.* (2020)

| Hacking the Hospital Environment | Healthcare | Not mentioned | Not mentioned | Designing youth-friendly hospital environments for satisfaction and better health outcomes 42 h | 27 young adults: students in architecture, design, engineering, communication and anthropology cancer patients | Effective mode of youth participation | Boisen *et al.* (2015) |
| Rehabilitation Hackathon | Healthcare | 2015/2016 | Harvard | First-ever rehabilitation hackathon In cooperation with MIT Hacking Medicine To accelerate and improve healthcare solutions and provide an educational experience for participants 2 days | 102 hackers, 19 physicians and other players in the ecosystem of rehabilitation and healthcare | Defining healthcare hackathons for internal and external stakeholders Explaining the hackathon process to internal and external stakeholders in a common language (taxonomy) Inviting participants, sponsors and collaborators who are interested in the topic | Silver *et al.* (2016) |

(Continued)

Table 1. (*Continued*)

Name	Industry	Date	Venue	Topic/Background	Participants	Lessons learned	Source
						Preparing written agreements that describe the expectations and deliverables for all participating organisations	
						Selecting metrics, collecting data and analysing the results of the hackathon	
						Anticipating concerns, particularly from academic physicians and scientists, about the potential for conflicts of interest and assisting them in avoiding these issues	
						Identifying relevant policies on intellectual property and conveying the policies to all participants	

e.Braun/ASiT Hackathon	Healthcare	2019	Belfast ASiT Conference	To generate productive, cross-speciality collaboration, as well as to solve current problems in healthcare 24-h event	Not mentioned	Not mentioned	Clements *et al.* (2019)
Iron Hack	Healthcare	2019	Florida	A rare disease-focused hackathon Symposium structure with methods presentations by experts and guest speakers To develop projects and ideas to visualise data, build databases, improve the diagnosis of rare diseases and study rare disease inheritance	Not mentioned	Cross-disease application of the results (can be applied to other rare diseases or general bioinformatics problems) Narrowing the focus (on individual cases of disease) improves the quality of outcomes	Ferreira *et al.* (2019)

(Continued)

Table 1. (*Continued*)

Name	Industry	Date	Venue	Topic/Background	Participants	Lessons learned	Source
International Meeting on Emerging Diseases and Surveillance Hackathon 2016	Healthcare	2016	Vienna	To develop solutions for intersection of emerging infectious diseases and climate change The MIT model was used again	100 participants Physicians, public health practitioners, veterinarians, IT professionals, engineers and entrepreneurs	Post-event: follow-up awards and encouraging teams to improve and develop their ideas Guaranteeing access to mentors and communication between teams (via discussion forums, mailing lists and others) Property rights: accessible and distributed to teams	Ramatowski *et al.* (2017)

| mHealth Colombia by SANA, Local Academia and ICT Industry | Healthcare | 2015 | Columbia | One week-long mHealth bootcamp and hackathon To develop mobile solutions for healthcare problems specific to the Columbian ecosystem Motivated by interest of the Colombian government in innovating processes in healthcare and ICT | More than 70 participants 18 interdisciplinary teams Advised by mentors from MIT, Massachusetts General Hospital — Harvard Medical School and local universities | It is useful to integrate education experts in the hackathon process to maximise the lessons from these events Clinical experts are important in the process to support and teach the participants The integration of high school students was rated as beneficial because they bring enthusiasm and motivation, foster the innovation process and influence the atmosphere positively | Angelidis et al. (2016) |

(Continued)

Table 1. *(Continued)*

Name	Industry	Date	Venue	Topic/Background	Participants	Lessons learned	Source
Hack for Youth	Healthcare	2015	Uganda	To design and develop technology solutions for adolescent sexual and reproductive health issues	80 participants from 17 countries	See mHealth Columbia	Angelidis *et al.* (2016)
mHealth Hackathon	Healthcare	2015	Greece	Identification of significant local healthcare problems and development of solutions based on open-source mHealth technology	Health scientists, innovators and engineers guided students	See mHealth Columbia	Angelidis *et al.* (2016)
mHealth Hackathon by Sana and Tecnologico de Monterrey in Mexico City	Healthcare	2016	Mexico	Topic selected by local physicians and researchers due to challenges facing elder care over the next years To develop mobile health solutions to address the growing needs of the elderly population	75 participants 11 multidisciplinary teams Telecommunication and computing engineers, biotechnologists, high school students, social workers and geriatricians	See mHealth Columbia	Angelidis *et al.* (2016)

In total, 11 articles about hackathons in healthcare were identified; most of them used the MIT Hacking Medicine model as a supportive framework for the organisation, followed by hackathons in technology, with 8 articles. The relatively large number of hackathons in healthcare is due to the search strategy, as PubMed was used. Furthermore, fewer hackathons that were scientifically evaluated were found in urban development, education, culture, environment, farming, research and Media.

To summarise the results, we link the lessons learned to three stages of a hackathon:

(1) **Pre-hackathon stage:** In this phase, the organisers should inform participants about the topics, techniques (e.g. for collaboration) as well as technologies offered during the event. According to MIT Hacking Medicine, it is especially important to be aware of relevant (in this case medical) innovations prior to the hackathon as this leads to increased efficiency.

To define the topic, we have to pay attention to the fact that narrowing the focus improves the quality of the outcome. Positive group dynamics can influence the event's outcomes. Groups should have a maximum of four to six members and consider a gender and expertise balance. To ensure productive cooperation as well as an optimal know-how exchange, we recommend including more experienced participants and enthusiastic students. Increasing diversity among participants would lead to greater creativity. Gender and expertise balance in teams has a positive effect. The distribution of roles within the groups should be promoted with appropriate strategies and mentoring to enable a sound distribution of work. Skill matching should also be considered, which means that the distribution of tasks should be based on the team members' skills and not only on their own interests. Social activities prior to the event can help the participants get to know each other better and promote their cooperation during the event. Team-building activities support collaboration and spark the development of innovative ideas.

Sponsors and collaborators who are interested in the topic of hackathon should be invited. Prominent members of the industry could be invited as jury members to evaluate the developed solutions.

At this stage, written agreements that describe the expectations and deliverables for all participating organisations should be prepared.

(2) **Operating stage:** Support of mentors, experts and organisers during the hackathon can influence the outcomes of the events.

At this stage, property rights should be accessible and distributed to teams and well-defined evaluation criteria should be provided.

The organisers should collect data during this phase to be able to analyse the results of the hackathon.

As prises foster motivation, offering rewards to the participants can be an effective approach. Integrating famous personalities in the jury can also motivate hackers and improve outcomes.

(3) **Post-hackathon stage:** The development of ideas should be promoted even in the following 3–6 months after the hackathon to move on with improving the original ideas. Examples of fostering motivation and participation are special follow-up awards, investor networking, access to mentors and communication between teams (through discussion forums, mailing lists and others).

4. What Makes VIENNO Hackathons Different from Others?

VIENNO involves structural, organisational, networking and cultural dimensions. It shows how to establish an innovation management framework by exploiting the highest level of potential of the public sector, corporations, universities and society. Its structural and organisational dimension has enabled healthcare organisations in Vienna to work together in the best possible manner to strengthen the entire healthcare system. Using this model in healthcare offers the opportunity to engage different partners, such as scientists, engineers, clinicians and patients (i.e. customers) in earlier stages of the innovation management process to produce substantial mutual benefits. The VIENNO innovation model is a platform where all the relevant stakeholders have a role to play.

What differentiates VIENNO from other hackathons?

(1) **Innovation ecosystem:** VIENNO strengthens the capacity of organisations, communities, institutions and systems through an innovation ecosystem that activates the major players. This established ecosystem provides a solid starting point for the hackathons. The interconnected members of the ecosystem are familiar with the complex issues in their field. Thus, the hackathon topic need not be explained to the participants and, consequently, they can proceed with addressing the issue quickly.

Furthermore, the VIENNO ecosystem is constructed such that diversity in expertise in the community is an inherent fit for hackathons. The interests, experiences, skills and knowledge of the community members are known, which also allows an optimal composition of teams for hackathons.

(2) **Cultural dimension:** VIENNO creates a network that covers the key players shaping the concerned sector. The members of this network collaborate to realise innovation solutions for their common challenges in various ways. Social innovation events, such as Inno-day 2020 under the motto "Innovation = Shaping the Future Together" at the General Hospital of Vienna to honour the innovators of the hospital and VAMED-KMB along with a cabaret show promote cooperation among community members. The continuity of these programmes connects people and strengthens community cohesion. This approach emphasises how VIENNO prepares the ground for a successful start in the hackathons.

(3) **Holistic system:** In VIENNO, the hackathons do not appear like a short pulse, nor are they standalone events that take place detached from institutional structures, without any connection to a larger whole. VIENNO treats hackathons as an integral component of an entire system. This philosophy enables VIENNO to organise hackathons with less effort because much of the prerequisites to run successful hackathons (pre-stage and post-stage) exist in the system.

(4) **Shared awareness:** In VIENNO, each individual node is mindful of the whole system. This shared awareness allows for fast, flexible and

smooth coordination and decision-making, which are far more adaptive and co-creative than any other model currently being used in major organisations. VIENNO and its eco-systemic fundamentals ensure that right innovation initiatives will be successfully created. VIENNO ensures that the hackathons generate reliable results that are not left to chance.

To summarise, the great organisational effort for classic hackathons and the unpredictable factors involved can be effectively managed by the established structures of VIENNO and the often-uncertain quality of results in hackathons can become considerably more reliable due to this ecosystem.

5. What Will the Future of Healthcare Be Like?

The healthcare system is subject to enormous changes. Precision medicine, legal regulations, technical developments and social change are just a few examples of the factors that drive the shift in this sector. The known trend towards economisation of medicine, an undesirable development in some aspects, is losing its appeal because of the COVID-19 pandemic. Coping with current and future challenges due to the increasingly severe consequences of the pandemic leads to the development and uptake of innovative solutions that address the needs of today's crisis management.

Creativity and professionalism are necessary to manage this change and the challenges facing the healthcare system, especially in using instruments to meet the new circumstances.

By applying VIENNO to manage the uncertainties and unpredictabilities related to the classic hackathons, this instrument can be an effective way for large organisations to deliver breakthrough innovations at start-up speed. VIENNO hacks the old processes focusing on a concrete output in its cross-functional structure by fostering a patient-centric and can-do culture.

Therefore, VIENNO hackathons provide a sound basis to develop solutions for the manifold future demands faced by the healthcare sector.

References

Angelidis, P., Berman, L., Casas-Perez, M. D. L. L., Celi, L. A., Dafoulas, G. E., Dagan, A., … & Otine, C. (2016) The hackathon model to spur innovation around global mHealth. *Journal of Medical Engineering & Technology*, 40(7–8), 392–399.

Boisen, K. A., Boisen, A., Thomsen, S. L., Matthiesen, S. M., Hjerming, M. & Hertz, P. G. (2015) Hacking the hospital environment: Young adults designing youth-friendly hospital rooms together with young people with cancer experiences. *International Journal of Adolescent Medicine and Health*, 29(4), e20150072.

Briscoe, G. (2014) Digital innovation: The hackathon phenomenon.

Charvat, K., Bye, B. L., Mildorf, T., Berre, A. J. & Jedlicka, K. (2018) Open data, VGI and citizen observatories INSPIRE hackathon. *International Journal of Spatial Data Infrastructures Research*, 13, 109–130.

Clements, J. M., Humm, G. & Nally, D. M. (2020) Innovation in surgical practice. In: *The Association of Surgeons in Training Conference — Belfast 2019*.

De Winne, J., Filipan, K., Moens, B., Devos, P., Leman, M., Botteldooren, D. & De Coensel, B. (2020) The soundscape hackathon as a methodology to accelerate co-creation of the urban public space. *Applied Sciences*, 10(6), 1932.

Ferreira, G. C., Oberstaller, J., Fonseca, R., Keller, T. E., Adapa, S. R., Gibbons, J., … & Dayhoff II, G. W. (2019) Iron Hack — A symposium/hackathon focused on porphyrias, Friedreich's ataxia, and other rare iron-related diseases. F1000Research, 8.

Gabrilove, J. L., Backeris, P., Lammers, L., Costa, A., Fattah, L., Eden, C., … & Costa, K. (2018) 2527 Mount Sinai health hackathon: Harnessing the power of collaboration to advance experiential team science education. *Journal of Clinical and Translational Science*, 2(Suppl 1), 58.

Giffard-Roisin, S., Gagne, D., Boucaud, A., Kégl, B., Yang, M., Charpiat, G. & Monteleoni, C. (2018, September) The 2018 climate informatics hackathon: Hurricane intensity forecast. In: *8th International Workshop on Climate Informatics*.

Green, B. N., Johnson, C. D. & Adams, A. (2006) Writing narrative literature reviews for peer-reviewed journals: Secrets of the trade. *Journal of Chiropractic Medicine*, 5(3), 101–117.

Haddaway, N. & Westgate M. J. (2018) *Evidence Synthesis Hackathon 2018*. Stockholm Environment Institute, Sweden, 31.

Jetzek, T. (2015) Elements of a successful Big Data hackathon in a smart city context. *Geoforum Perspektiv*, 14(25), 51–60.

Karlsen, J. & Løvlie, A. S. (2017) 'You can dance your prototype if you like': Independent filmmakers adapting the hackathon. *Digital Creativity*, 28(3), 224–239.

Lee, C. (2016) Health hackathons. *International Journal of Infectious Diseases*, 53, 7.

Maaravi, Y. (2018) Using hackathons to teach management consulting. *Innovations in Education and Teaching International*, 1–11.

Nolte, A., Pe-Than, E. P. P., Filippova, A., Bird, C., Scallen, S. & Herbsleb, J. D. (2018) You hacked and now what? — Exploring outcomes of a corporate hackathon. *Proceedings of the ACM on Human-Computer Interaction*, 2(CSCW), 1–23.

Olson, K. R., Walsh, M., Garg, P., Steel, A., Mehta, S., Data, S., … & Bangsberg, D. R. (2017) Health hackathons: Theatre or substance? A survey assessment of outcomes from healthcare-focused hackathons in three countries. *BMJ Innovations*, 3(1), 37–44.

Pogačar, K. & Žižek, A. (2016) Urban hackathon–alternative information based and participatory approach to urban development. *Procedia Engineering*, 161, 1971–1976.

Purwanto, A., Zuiderwijk, A. & Janssen, M. (2019, September) Citizens' motivations for engaging in open data hackathons. In: *International Conference on Electronic Participation*. Springer, Cham, pp. 130–141.

Ramatowski, J. W., Lee, C. X., Mantzavino, A., Ribas, J., Guerra, W., Preston, N. D., … & Lassmann, B. (2017) Planning an innovation marathon at an infectious disease conference with results from the International Meeting on Emerging Diseases and Surveillance 2016 Hackathon. *International Journal of Infectious Diseases*, 65, 93–97.

Sadr, M. & Granig, P. (2019) From ego to eco: What has VIENNO–the Vienna Innovation Model–got to do with it? In: *ISPIM Conference Proceedings*. The International Society for Professional Innovation Management (ISPIM), pp. 1–8.

Schulze, S. K., Ramšak, Ž., Hoang, Y., Zdravevski, E., Pfeil, J., Duarte López, A., … & Zagoršcak, M. (2018) *Proceedings of the "Think Tank Hackathon"*, Big Data Training School for Life Sciences Follow-Up, Ljubljana, 6th–7th February 2018. EMBnet.journal, 24, 1–4.

Sherman, A. T., Oliva, L., Golaszewski, E., Phatak, D., Scheponik, T., Herman, G. L., … & Bard, G. V. (2019) The CATS hackathon: Creating and refining test items for cybersecurity concept inventories. *IEEE Security & Privacy*, 17(6), 77–83.

Shin, N., Vela, K. & Evans, K. (2020) The research role of the librarian at a community health hackathon — A technical report. *Journal of Medical Systems*, 44(2), 36.

Silver, J. K., Binder, D. S., Zubcevik, N. & Zafonte, R. D. (2016) Healthcare hackathons provide educational and innovation opportunities: A case study and best practice recommendations. *Journal of Medical Systems*, 40(7), 177.

Suominen, A. H., Halvari, S. & Jussila, J. (2019) World heritage meets smart city in an urban-educational hackathon in Rauma. *Technology Innovation Management Review*, 9(9), 44–53.

Theise, A. (2017) Open cultural data hackathon coding Da Vinci — Bring the digital commons to life.

Valjamae, A., Evers, L., Allison, B. Z., Ongering, J., Riccio, A., Igardi, I. & Lamas, D. (2017, March) The BrainHack project: Exploring art-BCI hackathons. In: *Proceedings of the 2017 ACM Workshop on an Application-Oriented Approach to BCI Out of the Laboratory*, pp. 21–24.

Wang, J. K., Roy, S. K., Barry, M., Chang, R. T. & Bhatt, A. S. (2018) Institutionalizing healthcare hackathons to promote diversity in collaboration in medicine. *BMC Medical Education*, 18(1), 269.

Webb, H., Nurse, J. R., Bezuidenhout, L. & Jirotka, M. (2019, May) Lab hackathons to overcome laboratory equipment shortages in Africa: Opportunities and challenges. In: *Extended Abstracts of the 2019 CHI Conference on Human Factors in Computing Systems*, pp. 1–8.

Chapter 5

Speeding Up Innovative Solutions Development in Emergencies: Lessons Learned from the Inspire Ventilator Project

Ana Paula P. Leme Barbosa[*,‡], Ana Lucia F. Facin[†,§],
and Mario S. Salerno[*,¶]

[*]Production Engineering Department,
Polytechnic School, University of São Paulo (USP), Brazil

[†]Production Engineering Department,
Paulista University, São Paulo State University (UNESP), Brazil

[‡]aleme@usp.br
[§]affacin@gmail.com
[¶]msalerno@usp.br

The COVID-19 pandemic brought challenges to society, demanding local and innovative solutions due to the lack of international suppliers. In Brazil, led by the University of Sao Paulo, an emergency pulmonary mechanical ventilation equipment, cheaper than the existing equipment, was developed in a month to be manufactured by local industries, involving 40 multidisciplinary researchers and companies from different sectors. The ability to create this solution articulated by several actors in a small amount of time and with limited resources led us to study this case as an opportunity to learn and be well prepared to face other turbulent contexts. We found that a multidisciplinary knowledge-intense network provided the ground where orchestrators emerged. These orchestrators assumed roles that were not part of their job but were part of their skills. They worked together, taking the roles related to their network and skills. With their legitimacy within the organisation and within society, these orchestrators, leveraged by the communication of a clear mission, fostered access to knowledge and other resources. This chapter briefly describes the case and provides some reflections about the roles augmented for turbulent times, the embedded network, and the orchestrators' skills throughout the innovation journey.

1. Introduction

One of the main challenges brought about by the COVID-19 pandemic is the lack of global supplies to meet the demand for essential resources to treat infected people. This shortage is worse in large countries with under-developed industrial infrastructure, such as Brazil. This very atypical situation demanded local and innovative solutions. The mechanical ventilation equipment components were among the most requested and bottlenecked. Suppliers of such devices directed their sales to more prosperous countries. Besides, restrictions in components supply caused a reduction in local production. There was an urgent need to develop and produce pulmonary ventilators locally to circumvent the scarcity of imported components. It would need to be fast since the death toll mounted daily. To quickly meet such massive restrictions, the ventilator developed should meet some design criteria: be simple, effective and safe enough to be approved by the Regulatory Agency. The case we select to study is how to speed up product development to face emergencies. The context is specific, but we expect that the insights can be more broadly applied, especially to help build faster responses in emergencies in any place.

The new context of unprecedented challenges, extreme time pressure, in which the point is to save lives, makes it necessary to go beyond generating and capturing value. It is different from the 'normal' innovation-driven environment that innovation management theorists (Bagno *et al.*, 2017; Gomes *et al.*, 2018; O'Connor, 2008, O'Connor *et al.*, 2018; Salerno *et al.*, 2015) call a dynamic or turbulent environment.

Such unique challenges brought about by the pandemic demand efficiency and even faster organisational adaptation like to be strategy-oriented (to find a suitable solution), to give quick responses (because, in this case, time is life, not money), to be economical (due to the supplies shortage), and to be flexible (to deal with the mishaps).

Having the necessary capabilities to mobilise and orchestrate the required competencies and resources is essential for success, mainly in developing complex and knowledge-intensive projects, which is the case of products related to the health industry.

The innovativeness of the case is the ability to quickly develop a complex and knowledge-intensive product, with resource restriction, and finally achieving a much lower price than the available products in the market. Moreover, the device was developed within and coordinated by a university, not by an incumbent or startup as expected. Therefore, it is an opportunity to understand how it all happened to identify specific ways of management that could enhance the new product development in an emergency context.

Hence, based on this case, we aim to answer the question: How to successfully develop a new product in a context of extreme resource and time constraints?

To achieve our goal, we explored two concepts that were at the centre of the narrative of the participants of the project:

 (i) Network building, which describes how the access and integration of the participants of the project occurred, helping to develop the project and leveraging the knowledge base quickly;
(ii) Orchestrator roles and capabilities to describe the roles and capabilities required to accelerate the project development.

We emphasise that observing and monitoring this peculiar and unique case provided the identification of some lessons learned on how to innovate in extreme emergencies; however, the findings were not from extensive research. Thus, it is also an opportunity for future studies.

To provide a better idea of the process of our study, we organised the chapter as follows: first, we describe the method used and, in the result section, we present the concepts and discuss the findings; later, we offer the implications. The reader may expect a better clarification of the concepts priorly; however, the study followed an inductive approach. We started with a broad research question, and the core themes (network and orchestration) emerged during the interviews and data analysis.

2. Methods

We employed a qualitative research approach for helping identify critical factors that emerged from the case that could give a new answer to a complex context. Then we discussed these crucial factors through the lens of the existing literature. In this research, we adopted an interpretative approach as we are interested in understanding the project development process from the perspective of the project participants. We discuss the critical factors for the project development from the informants' view after describing the case organised as a traditional product development process to facilitate reading comprehension.

We began data collection from the very beginning of the project. The data starts at the call for projects that could face challenges related to COVID-19 (internal documents, emails) and followed the whole project development (that was a fast-pacing innovation project) through documents and interviews. The interview data include non-structured interviews with the project participants (project leaders and project team members), an external participant and the Dean of the School responsible for the project. The documents include emails shared by the University's professors, the project website, news (broadcast media broadly covered the project, local newspapers, and the University Press), speeches of team members (recorded) and informal interviews with team members. We recorded some interviews, and some of them relied on researcher notes.

We conducted the interviews in a narrative mode. Participants first told their story about the project from its very beginning. Then, we asked the interviewee to give further details about specific information that emerged during the interview. We could thus focus further on parts of their stories when critical factors emerged. We initially identified project participants through an internal newsletter shared with faculty members and news media. Then, we moved to theoretical sampling based on the factors that emerged from documents and interviews, aligned with the grounded-theory approach (Glaser *et al.*, 1968).

We selected and analysed data to label the direct statements through an open-coding approach (Strauss and Corbin, 2008). The coding focus was on the critical factors identified in informants' speeches. Two researchers individually identified the vital factors and then compared and discussed to verify if they were analytically distinct. The factors considered decisive for the success in quickly developing the project, presented in all or most of the interviews, were: (i) the support of the leaders enabling collaboration; (ii) the network orchestration roles to search and access resources; (iii) individuals' network; (iv) common identity and mission; (v) the focal actor reputation.

The next step was defining core concepts common to all the factors, representing an overarching concept encompassing the whole project. This definition occurred by a comparison between the issues that emerged as critical factors for network mobilisation.

3. Results

3.1. The case: Inspire — an emergency ventilator development

At the centre of this case is a University, the most prominent Public University in the country (the University of Sao Paulo, from now on called USP), which has Schools in several knowledge areas. At the beginning of the pandemic, the University leaders launched an internal call asking for solutions that could help the Brazilian society face the pandemic.

Immediately, the consensus on starting a study to verify the feasibility of developing an emergency mechanical ventilator in Brazil using local suppliers took place at a meeting of the Engineering School leaders, who also decided to establish several fronts to combat the COVID-19 pandemic. The mechanical ventilator project was a 'natural' project to support because there was an experienced Professor in the field who, together with researchers from the Medical School, has dedicated over 18 years to studying lung physiology and medical equipment.

At that time, Prof. Raúl Gonzalez Lima (from now on called Prof. Raúl), the experienced Professor from the Engineering School, was invited to lead this study. He took on the challenge because he was 'already convinced that although the regulatory process was very long, it was worth trying to make the emergency ventilator due to the humanitarian crisis that promised to be very dramatic if there were no such ventilators available in Brazil'. Suddenly, a race against time was triggered to access the necessary knowledge and resources and to integrate all efforts to quickly make ventilators available to the hospitals, which would soon have an enormous need for this equipment.

Fortunately, the project team accomplished the challenge due to the joint effort of a large number of collaborators led by the Engineering School, involving about 40 multidisciplinary researchers, multi-sector companies, open-source communities and donors who participated through crowdfunding platforms. The remarkable work done by this group made it possible to design, in a month, a 15-times-less-expensive solution to be subsequently tested and manufactured by another set of players (e.g. Brazilian Navy and research institutes) quickly brought together.

3.1.1. *Starting the mission*

Faced with this great challenge, right after the leadership project call, Prof. Raúl quickly sketched an initial diagram of how the equipment could be. From this diagram, he started to identify the needs for an initial team, and what types of specialists would be needed. However, this team grew in a not very controlled way, and in the first two weeks of the project, the team already had 40 specialists from different areas of knowledge. Throughout the project, it became much more significant. In this case, the existing relations with other USP units were fundamental. The articulation among them occurred initially in a very spontaneous way. The people who have been initially involved began to search through their contacts for the specialities necessary throughout the project. As stated by Liedi Legi Bariani Bernucci, the Faculty Dean, 'it was a chain that helped spontaneously, it was a very supportive movement' and also by Dario Gramorelli, the technical leader, 'suddenly, there were dozens of people involved from different areas'. It is worth mentioning that there is no established process in the organisation for articulating multidisciplinary research projects of any nature; there is a collaboration between units, but each one independently articulates and seeks its partnerships depending on the needs for each research. In other words, there is no institutional process for orchestrating these initiatives to seek competencies within the university.

3.1.2. *Fuzzy front end and prototyping*

At the beginning of the project, the project team resolved the uncertainties more quickly and opened the project to a vast network of collaborators, companies and individuals. They started to contribute to resolving the problems that arose during the design of the product. The project team established that the collaboration should follow some design principles, clearly defined by the project team to meet project restrictions regarding time and resources. Some examples of these restrictions were ease of manufacturing and distribution, using the minimum possible number of imported components, and more importantly, ensuring the minimum necessary characteristics that would allow its approval by the Regulatory Agency.

The idea of having an open-source project from the beginning was to have people working in parallel on the project ('makers'). It helped make faster decisions by multiplying efforts to search for alternatives and make it possible to know if they were viable or discardable quickly. Thus, it helped to mitigate significant uncertainties faster. This community participation was intense, mainly in the prototyping phase. In a few days, the initial project idea evolved in the form of successive prototyping cycles (builds, tests and evaluates), implemented very quickly until it became a 'minimum viable product' that was already working with its most basic functionalities.

'Community Engagement' function was the most critical role in this project phase, mainly due to the adopted open-source character, which synchronised the collaboration of the community with what was being developed by the multidisciplinary team of specialists formed within the University. The role of this function was mainly one of mediation and encouragement. The project team used certain strict design principles to select the numerous solutions and alternatives the community offered. In this context, even the ideas that proved to be 'not feasible' helped to base the decisions and confirm that the following path was correct.

The project team assumed as indispensable some of these design principles such as price, safety and especially the time required to assemble and test the equipment. For example, they ruled out using components manufactured by 3D printers because it requires a longer manufacturing time compared to other types of more traditional processes. Numerous design decisions helped to make the product cheaper due to making several simplifications to the mechanical ventilator commonly produced by the industry while still ensuring it fulfilled its role robustly and safely, thus producing an elegant design from this point of view. As explained by Prof. Raúl, 'we had to think about a solution made by off-the-shelf components, and if possible, by Brazilian manufacturers. The reason is that supply chains were at risk of being broken, as happened a few weeks later, and it would be good to use several components that the Brazilian Regulatory Agency had already approved to minimise the regulatory problem'.

3.1.3. *Development*

To test the mechanism for controlling the dynamic response of the solution, the project team relied on a dynamic artificial lung test bench. One of the research labs within the University has this test bench. The project team had access to it to carry out the necessary tests, thus ensuring the required safety before carrying out clinical trials. These tests were fundamental to adjusting the ventilator control algorithm until this device met all the reactions expected. It is worth mentioning that during the bench testing phase, specialists from a government institution installed within the University campus, which is the Institute of Technological Research of the State of São Paulo (IPT), were also involved.

During the development phase, the project team acquired the necessary expertise to take care of legal and regulatory aspects. In this matter, the involvement of specialists from the Law School was fundamental. At that time, a focal figure emerged in the project, Dr Marcelo Knörish Zuffo, a Full Professor of the Electrical Engineering Department, to address these issues and give the project an institutional character. He orchestrated the actions that would complement the more technical role of Prof. Raúl. This articulation was also fundamental to activating the supply chain partners to produce and distribute the equipment.

3.1.4. *Testing*

In the clinical testing phase, the project team requested the participation of the Medical School, with its specialists represented from the beginning of the project, and also the Veterinary Medicine School, which was responsible for animal tests, carried out before tests with humans.

On the manufacturing side of the project, the University and the Brazilian Navy formed a production partnership. The production time is approximately 2 hours, and the estimated cost is 15 times less than the cost of commercial ventilators for each piece of equipment.

3.2. *The critical factors*

The Inspire project followed the classical new product development macro process but at a fast pace, which does not mean doing the same activities faster. Actually, it was an ad-hoc project, with no prior new product development formal process. We tried to understand factors related to the project governance that helped the project move forward

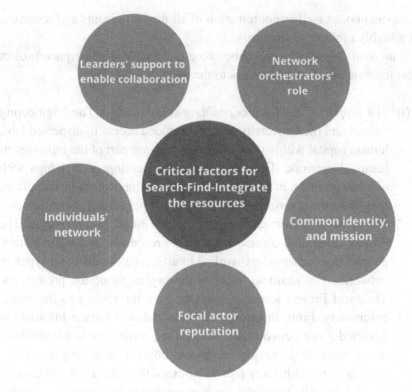

Figure 1.   Critical factors for network mobilisation.

quickly. In this section, we highlight some factors that emerged from the data we collected. Figure 1 summarises these factors.

About 30 days elapsed from the starting date on which the University's Board demanded solutions for COVID-19-related challenges until the trial in humans. The technical solution was not obvious and required an intense learning process involving several high-level specialists in the multidisciplinary fields and open-source platforms for parallel development. The main challenge was the pressure of time as if the solution took longer, it would not achieve the main objective of saving lives during the pandemic. The problems related to such a complex objective are, for example, accessing the knowledge dispersed within the network (search/find the knowledge and combine it) and the needed resources (such as labs, equipment components), as well as coordination of all the participants and resources in a highly productive rhythm.

In what follows, we describe some factors for the fast pace project development that fostered access to the needed resources:

(i) *The support of the leaders enabling collaboration*: The Engineering School and the University leaders provided access to dispersed labs, human capital within the Colleges, which are part of the intra-organisational network. They also helped to develop partnerships with external partners. In the current language of Innovation Management, they were the sponsors of the project that helped access resources.

(ii) *The network orchestration roles to search and access resources*: The project demanded diverse knowledge, resources, tasks and critical people; the orchestrators worked to articulate the different types of networks. For example, right at the beginning of the project, the Technical Project leader decided to open the project to the whole community. From this point, all widely shared project information attracted a vast network of collaborators, companies and individuals in the intra- and inter-organisational domain, resolving the uncertainties faster. Other key figures assumed the role of the orchestrator of other specific networks, such as a network for accessing external resources (financial, components) and a network for institutional matters, which assumed a more political role interacting with the Government and high-level suppliers. Besides, it is worth highlighting that collaboration with the project was voluntary, mission-oriented. There was one clear project leader but not one owner; it was a collaborative project.

(iii) *Individuals' network*: Participants joined the project without pre-assigned roles; those emerged during their activities. They brought their skills and resources, especially being able to orchestrate their network to access the needed resources. For example, one of the professors is embedded in an industry network, and he accessed resources from the corporate world. Thus, an orchestrator role emerged over the project, and the orchestrator became responsible for the activities related to the kind of network he was embedded in.

(iv) *Common identity and mission*: Universities encompass characteristics unique to this type of institution: a centre of knowledge with highly skilled professionals, diverse labs and resource types integrated by a common identity. Despite the diversity in terms of specialised knowledge that is not accessed regularly, all knowledge under the same leadership and identity facilitates new connections. Also, it eliminates bureaucracies that may exist with external partnerships when working in the intra-organisational domain.

(v) *The focal actor reputation*: The project's participants had to orchestrate several kings of resources with different types of individuals and organisations. For example, they have to access external partners that could help manufacture the product, taking on responsibilities that are not typical of a university. But due to the University's and the orchestrators' reputations, the orchestrators managed to attract several partners that were essential to enable the full-scale production of the ventilator.

In summary, the case description illustrates the development of an innovative product in the context of the pandemic. We highlighted critical factors that were part of the informant's speeches. We extracted a common concept among them: the network mobilisation for identifying and integrating the resources for the new product development. In the next section, we discuss the findings.

4. Discussion and Implications

In the innovation field, network studies concern access to knowledge and complementary resources among a set of actors connected by a set of ties. The existing network fosters complementary knowledge closely related to the firm knowledge stock and, consequently, related to exploitative projects. In turn, the knowledge search may move beyond existing ties for explorative projects and challenge the firm's absorptive capacity, mainly in projects characterised by uncertainties and expertise not closely related to the firm's knowledge stock. Thus, the challenge is to find partners that are not so close that they could not provide the needed knowledge, but also not too far that they could harm mutual understanding (Gilsing *et al.*,

2008). Hence, the cognitive distance discussion in the network and innovation literature takes place.

Apart from cognitive distance, new knowledge sources are also a key research issue for innovation. In this case, the discussion is on the structural aspects of the network. When the connection is across groups, there is a more significant opportunity to create new combinations of knowledge (Burt, 2004) and, consequently, to foster exploration projects. However, the possibility to develop such ties is affected by the position of the actor within the network, which means that a more central position favours access to network activity and fosters connections with new groups (Gilsing *et al.*, 2008).

However, the network by itself does not develop a project. There is a need for articulation, which means there is a need for people taking action to find and integrate the needed knowledge and other resources, the ones that aim to be part of the project, and the ones that have the skills and expertise for each phase of the project (O'Connor *et al.*, 2018). Building strong and diverse network ties could help meet innovation goals, and in general, in dynamic or turbulent environments, strengthening existing partnerships is more conducive to firm innovation (Yang *et al.*, 2021).

In our study case, the Engineering School took on the central position in the network. Some members of the Engineering School assumed the role of facilitators–orchestrators with neutrality and integrity, which are typical characteristics of this type of orchestrator (Hurmelinna-Laukkanen and Nätti, 2018). These characteristics were fundamental to fostering engagement in the innovation network from the beginning of the project, and a good university reputation may have facilitated this engagement.

Our findings reinforce what Tidd and Bessant (2020) highlight about the power of innovation networks to compensate for resource limitations. Our results also support the notion that creating appropriate structures and behaviours for developing effective innovation management using networks is imperative. For example, to access the necessary resources, it is interesting to keep 'high levels of informality to build on a shared vision and rapid decision-making but possibly to build network linkages' (Tidd and Bessant, 2020, p. 60).

As highlighted by Diamond and Vangen (2017), 'attempts to innovate without changing underlying or rigid structures, processes and behaviours are unlikely to be effective', and added that effective collaborative innovation is a process 'dependent on context and resulting from shared understandings and actions of the participants'. In this sense, having strong relational skills and coordination abilities facilitates the adoption of flexible structures (Anser *et al.*, 2020).

Tidd and Bessant (2020) point out some challenges in managing innovation networks to construct the appropriate structures and have expected behaviours, such as establishing fundamental operation processes to deal with knowledge management, information flow management, motivation and coordination.

These activities call for orchestration (Hurmelinna-Laukkanen and Nätti, 2018) and were conducted, in our case, by more than one person, each of them with a specific role, which we discuss as follows.

Some specific activities could require that orchestrators take different roles and sometimes adopt unnatural roles (Hurmelinna-Laukkanen and Nätti, 2018). Our study found that orchestrators' augmented role capabilities (Figure 2) favoured speeding up uncertainty mitigation, access to resources and project development. These orchestrators could take atypical roles to deal with the sudden emergence of opportunities or threats that demanded actions. They went beyond the typical activities of the University, which is to act mainly in the fuzzy front end and on the early concepts and design principles. Their action spread over the initial development to other phases, such as production feasibility, equipment

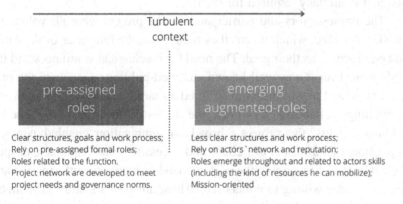

Turbulent context

pre-assigned roles

emerging augmented-roles

Clear structures, goals and work process;
Rely on pre-assigned formal roles;
Roles related to the function.
Project network are developed to meet project needs and governance norms.

Less clear structures and work process;
Rely on actors´network and reputation;
Roles emerge throughout and related to actors skills (including the kind of resources he can mobilize);
Mission-oriented

Figure 2.   The emerging augmented roles in a turbulent context.

approval, partnership for manufacturing, distribution and training people to use it at the hospitals properly.

The role-augmentation capability involves 'sensing the need to take action, but also go much deeper: the orchestrator needs to alter its characteristics, its position, or goals (at least temporarily)' (Hurmelinna-Laukkanen and Nätti, 2018, p. 75). We found some roles adopted by the orchestrators in later stages, such as ensuring testing safety, norms adequacy and reaching high-capacity suppliers to manufacture the ventilator, which are roles not expected in the research or education domain of the University. In the initial phase of the project, when rapid prototyping occurred with the parallel development of technology solutions (e.g. accessing open-source knowledge hubs), the orchestrators assumed the roles of agenda setting and mobilisation to get the network members working towards the same goal and to motivate collaboration and clarify goals, respectively (Hurmelinna-Laukkanen and Nätti, 2018). In the later stages, the orchestrators assumed other roles to provide access to resources dispersed over the University (labs, multidisciplinary knowledge, *in vivo* testing) and develop a network to address the production supply and regulation issues.

These different roles and skills, which emerge according to the innovation stages, can be compared to the innovation function characteristics described by O'Connor *et al.* (2018). Yet, in this case, there is no predefined role or function. The role or function emerged during the process by the action of individuals that had the needed knowledge, network position and legitimacy required for the role.

The orchestrators and participants of the project were all voluntary, mission-oriented, which means they recognised the relevance of the cause and embraced it as their goal. The need for mechanical ventilators and the USP project for it was well-known and well-publicised, as were the project design and requirements. It fostered a shared vision over the network, facilitating collaboration within the network to access the needed resources. Thus, the project's broad communication enabled people's engagement (Barbosa *et al.*, 2020) and access to some resources, despite the challenge of managing the high demand of media for information and diverse people willing to collaborate. Thus, this case illustrates the mobilisation of a network for developing a product during a pandemic context.

We highlight the emergence of a role-augmented perspective associated with the innovation function role in a knowledge-intensive network and a mission-oriented project for this development. This innovation role was developed aligned with the idea that major innovation requires different competencies according to the project phase, which is associated with each person's skills (O'Connor *et al.*, 2018).

The network characteristics helped access resources for some of the following reasons — first, the easy access to complementary knowledge. Second, the existence of a common language within the network (even when cognitive distance exists in the domain area, there is a common understanding of how to work due to the background of the professionals involved in researching and solving complex problems). Finally, the project relevance for society (which developed a mission-oriented project and a shared and clear goal). Additionally, the leadership of core people who augmented their roles and mobilised others made the project happen.

4.1. *Implications for theory and future research*

We expect this study to contribute to managing innovative solutions to face turbulent contexts, especially regarding network antecedents and orchestration roles.

During normal times, the innovation function is responsible for systematising the innovation (O'Connor *et al.*, 2008). It has a critical role of resource orchestration, with specific skills and expertise according to the phase of the strategic innovation process (O'Connor *et al.*, 2018). However, during emergencies, we notice that some roles of innovation function emerged from diverse parts of the organisation. We do not identify a pre-defined innovation function in the studied case, but it emerged as a role-augmenting capability (Hurmelinna-Laukkanen and Nätti, 2018). Thus, this idea of role-augmenting capability may be fruitful research for contexts of uncertainties in which people may assume responsibilities that are not part of their routines. For example, identifying the orchestrators for emergence contexts (which involves technical capability and leadership skills, network antecedents, legitimacy). How helpful would it be to have a previously established innovation function in turbulent times? Would the role-augment capability be a case applied only when there is no pre-defined innovation function? How to educate people to have the flexibility to assume other roles in turbulent contexts?

Moreover, the network the organisation (and its participants) is embedded in is a core factor to allow access to the needed resources that might overcome the unit or the organisation network. In normal times, the initial project team can build the network as part of project development. In turbulent times the existing network is where the resources will be accessed (there is not much time to develop new partnerships), as the parties already know each other. In this sense, enriching the network would be necessary for preparing the organisation for turbulent scenarios, even during normal times. Thus, establishing relationships within the organisation and knowledge centres (universities, research institutes) would help develop a network for collaboration in turbulent times. It can help build the knowledge of how to work together (essential to speeding up the project). Future studies in this matter can focus on understanding how to quickly establish and manage relationships within the organisation and with knowledge centres to facilitate collaboration in turbulent times. For example, does the existing governance structure facilitate collaboration? What kind of change in the governance structure is needed to allow establishing collaboration at a fast pace?

4.2. *Implication for policymaking*

The pandemic demonstrated the challenge of providing a quick response to a high-impact sanitary crisis — diverse actors of society developed projects to face it, from medical equipment to medicines and vaccines. However, emergent economies struggled to develop solutions, access the needed resources and provide disease control properly and in time. While more generally we identify a lack of coordination and network articulation, we suggest policies that intensify network connection between country universities and abroad, between universities and other actors based on this case study. This network needs to be built over the years, fostering relationships and learning about how to work together. Besides, orchestrators are vital levers for actions within the network. Their coordination enables integration and moves projects forward. In this sense, public policies could stimulate some key institutions to act as orchestrators and be prepared to assume this role in emergency scenarios, composing an innovation system for such scenarios. Initiatives should not depend on the occurrence of an emergency to foster this system development. Governments can develop projects focused on the country's social issues, which could have a broad impact on social welfare. We may be able to identify orchestrators and connections from such actions and expect them to be better coordinated when facing new emergencies.

4.3. *Future delivery/models*

Supposing that society faces extreme events in the future, the learnings from the COVID-19 pandemic could provide knowledge for succeeding in important projects by knowing how to orchestrate multiple heterogeneous actors in a scenario of time and resource restrictions.

This study provides examples of how to face constraints in a scenario of severe societal harm, being not an example exclusive for the ones that are at universities. It demonstrates the power of engaging people to solve a common problem with a clear set of objectives, despite its unclear path. Some requirements are to be known in advance by the team and others to discover on the fly and quickly articulate by accessing resources within the network or easily accessing network members. Thus, we provide a set of questions that can help managers and other professionals who want to contribute to solving fundamental challenges to think about:

- Are we immersed in a rich and diverse network with easy access to complementary knowledge?
- How can we engage in a diverse network if our daily lives are well set within a small number of well-known players?
- What roles can I assume that are not my direct job? Which is my augmented capability (or my company's augmented capability)?

These are some insights we provide to provoke the readers into thinking about how you or your company would be an essential player in a scenario of a societal crisis, such as the one we have faced in the health domain.

Additionally, learnings from this case study could inspire innovation management beyond crisis. For example, with fast-pacing technology development, projects are being developed in a less clear, less stable and less structured work environment. Thus, the work process may benefit from enabling people to operate with their skill sets rather than pre-defined roles. Companies may assess governance mechanisms that could foster such an approach. Moreover, network-building capability is a theme that companies should care more about, which is more than searching, finding and establishing partnerships; it involves learning how to collaborate and integrate the knowledge. Finally, the Inspire case shows an extraordinary engagement, with people searching for solutions as their primary reward. It sets a challenge for traditional companies: to find the proper human resources systems to incite people to auto mobilise themselves to act.

References

Anser, M. K., Yousaf, Z., Usman, M., Yousaf, S., Fatima, N., Hussain, H. & Waheed, J. (2020) Strategic business performance through network capability and structural flexibility. *Management Decision*, 59(2), 426–445. Available at: https://doi.org/10.1108/MD-06-2019-0741.

Bagno, R. B., Salerno, M. S. & Silva, D. O. (2017) Models with graphical representation for innovation management: A literature review. *R&D Management*, 47(4), 637–653. Available at: https://doi.org/10.1111/radm.12254.

Barbosa, A. P. P. L., Salerno, M. S., Brasil, V. C. & Nascimento, P. T. de S. (2020) Coordination approaches to foster open innovation R&D projects performance. *Journal of Engineering and Technology Management*, 58, 101603. Available at: https://doi.org/10.1016/j.jengtecman.2020.101603.

Burt, R. (2004) Structural holes and good ideas. *American Journal of Sociology*, 110(2), 349–399. Available at: https://doi.org/10.1086/421787.

Diamond, J. & Vangen, S. (2017) Coping with austerity: Innovation via collaboration or retreat to the known? *Public Money & Management*, 37(1), 47–54. Available at: https://doi.org/10.1080/09540962.2016.1249231.

Gilsing, V., Nooteboom, B., Vanhaverbeke, W., Duysters, G. & van den Oord, A. (2008) Network embeddedness and the exploration of novel technologies: Technological distance, betweenness centrality and density. *Research Policy*,

37(10), 1717–1731. Available at: https://doi.org/10.1016/j.respol.2008. 08.010.

Glaser, B. G., Strauss, A. L. & Strutzel, E. (1968) The discovery of grounded theory; strategies for qualitative research. *Nursing Research*, 17(4), 364.

Gomes, L. A. V., Facin, A. L. F., Salerno, M. S. & Ikenami, R. K. (2018) Unpacking the innovation ecosystem construct: Evolution, gaps, and trends. *Technological Forecasting and Social Change*, 136, 30–48. Available at: https://doi.org/10.1016/j.techfore.2016.11.009.

Hurmelinna-Laukkanen, P. & Nätti, S. (2018) Orchestrator types, roles and capabilities—A framework for innovation networks. *Industrial Marketing Management*, 74, 65–78. Available at: https://doi.org/10.1016/j.indmarman. 2017.09.020.

O'Connor, G. C. (2008) Major innovation as a dynamic capability: A system approach. *Journal of Product Innovation Management*, 25(4), 313–330. Available at: https://doi.org/10.1111/j.1540-5885.2008.00304.x.

O'Connor, G. C., Corbett, A. C. & Peters, L. S. (2018) *Beyond the Champion Institutionalizing Innovation Through People*. Stanford University Press.

O'Connor, G. C., Leifer, R., Paulson, A. S. & Peters, L. S. (2008) *Grabbing Lightning: Building a Capability for Breakthrough Innovation*. Jossey-Bass.

Salerno, M. S., Gomes, L. A. V., Silva, D. O., Bagno, R. B. & Freitas, S. L. T. U. (2015) Innovation processes: Which process for which project? *Technovation*, 35, 59–70.

Strauss, A. L. & Corbin, J. (2008) *Basics of Qualitative Research: Techniques and Procedures for Developing Grounded Theory*. Sage.

Tidd, J. & Bessant, J. R. (2020) *Managing Innovation: Integrating Technological, Market, and Organisational Change*. John Wiley & Sons.

Yang, J., Zhang, J. & Zeng, D. (2021) Scientific collaboration networks and firm innovation: The contingent impact of a dynamic environment. *Management Decision*. Ahead-of-print. Available at: https://doi.org/10.1108/MD-08-2020-1050.

Chapter 6

Technology-Enhanced Learning (TEL) Solutions for COVID-19: Use Cases from Torbay and South Devon NHS Foundation Trust (TSDFT)

Payal Ghatnekar[*], Matthew Halkes[†], and Nick Peres[‡]

Torbay and South Devon NHS Foundation Trust,
Digital Futures Lab, Horizon Centre, Torquay, UK

*payal.ghatnekar@nhs.net
†matthew.halkes@nhs.net
‡n.peres@nhs.net*

The COVID-19 pandemic has highlighted new and existing challenges for the delivery of healthcare staff training, medical students learning programmes, and meeting both COVID-19 and non-COVID-19 patient requirements. Healthcare systems globally have and continue to experience these challenges, including a severe backlog of clinical activity. Torbay hospital (NHS-UK) has previously existing knowledge in the technology sphere that has been applied to identify and resolve pandemic priorities and needs. Access to Technology-Enhanced Learning (TEL) tools and services has enabled Torbay in expanding and scaling up technologies to deliver solutions. Using the 'double-diamond' design thinking methodology process, multi-expert teams (clinicians, educators and TEL developers) worked together to address some of the pandemic challenges. As a result of the rapid innovation that Torbay has undertaken, several use cases have emerged which may be applicable to healthcare workers, medical students and patients, nationally and internationally. In this chapter, we describe factors that enabled innovation, our thoughts on sustainability of the interventions post-pandemic and limitations of the tools. The primary aim of our chapter is to encourage healthcare providers to establish discourse on the role of TEL innovation for meeting COVID-19 priorities and to help inform further opportunities for innovation in the NHS. Our intention is to encourage other healthcare providers to explore design thinking and generate their individual TEL use cases.

1. Introduction

1.1. *TEL in healthcare and COVID-19*

Technology-Enhanced Learning (TEL) is the use of a wide array of technologies in the field of education and training. Within healthcare, TEL can be used to describe online learning experiences, virtual conferencing software, games, simulation technologies such as Augmented Reality (AR), Virtual Reality (VR) or Extended Reality (XR) and educational software applications. TEL is documented to facilitate knowledge acquisition, improved decision-making and enhanced skill training (Guze, 2015).

TEL-based training is not a substitute for experiential learning through face-to-face encounters within real-world clinical environments, but provides a useful adjunct to traditional didactic classroom teaching, while offering some distinct advantages. For example, TEL affords users the opportunity to practise and learn within safe environments, where they can make errors without the real-world consequences associated with patient outcomes. TEL programmes can be customised to deliver more personalised, transformative learner experiences that can be accessed by students and staff in a repeatable manner, at times which are convenient to them (Baxendale, 2017).

TEL programmes are becoming a large part of healthcare education and training in the UK and worldwide. The use of TEL in medical education has grown rapidly as a variety of technologies continue to be adopted for the purpose of teaching (Baxendale, 2017; Osborne *et al.*, 2021). According to Madani *et al.* (2017), clinical environments are undergoing considerable shifts as healthcare providers have started to focus on patient safety, accountability, transparency and improvement of overall patient experience. The state of medical education is also changing rapidly, greatly influenced by evolution in healthcare environments, changing role of GPs, changes in patient expectations, advancement in science and research into pedagogical techniques (Guze, 2015). Current challenges of healthcare workforce training are to develop well-trained staff that treat patients empathetically and focus on improving the quality of patient experiences. Patients who are satisfied with the care they receive, are more likely to comply with treatment and management.

Innovation in TEL has resulted in the development of more realistic scenarios and improved learning opportunities (Grimwood and Snell, 2020). This innovation is made possible through effective relationships between healthcare workers and educators, technology developers and designers, academia and economic/market variables that are affected due to changes in societal requirements. As TEL evolves, it allows healthcare innovators the opportunity to put into practical application, new ideas and concepts from clinical practice, with the end goal of improving patients' experiences (Baxendale, 2017; Madani *et al.*, 2017). Madani *et al.* (2017) stress that often when thinking of innovation in healthcare the focus is on medical devices or hardware, however, iterative improvement of TEL experiences is also a form of healthcare innovation that will eventually have implications on methodology, practice and patient experience.

The COVID-19 pandemic has resulted in accelerated innovation across a range of TEL modalities in response to the serious disruption caused to medical education and healthcare workers' training (Goh and Sandars, 2020; Li *et al.*, 2020). Face-to-face attendance had come to a halt and students were forced to work remotely from home (Goh and Sandars, 2020). During these challenging times, medical schools and hospitals rapidly scaled up available learning technologies to meet the requirements of education and training. The pandemic brought to attention the importance of streamlining medical education, so that clinical educators can use their time effectively and students acquire the real-world clinical skills they require. At the same time, educators needed to ensure that there is no detrimental impact on the student's experience or quality of education (Madani *et al.*, 2017).

One of the critical challenges that presented itself has been replicating real-world patient experiences or clinical encounters virtually (Goh and Sandars, 2020). Immersive virtual simulations may be a good substitute (Osborne *et al.*, 2021) as immersive technologies (XR) can enable educators to teach students in virtual environments that mimic real-world situations. Such innovations must be investigated further as tools that can be used in adjunct to real-world clinical scenario training. However medical educators have encountered a series of issues such as availability of physical resources, technical support and available budget while delivering TEL for COVID-19. Additional stress was put on the system due to the nature of the pandemic, the toll it took on physical and mental well-being and the time constraints within which to scale up available technology.

In 2013, Health Education England (HEE) launched the TEL programme, with the aim to educate healthcare workforce through evidence-based technology. Better-trained and experienced healthcare workers are beneficial for patients, colleagues and the wider community. The Torbay Virtual Reality Lab & Digital Futures Programme (based at Torbay and South Devon NHS Foundation Trust (TSDFT), Torquay, Devon) was initially funded by HEE, to investigate emerging technologies to tackle challenges and the workforce digital literacy within the NHS, specifically in areas of medical education, digital workforce skills and where appropriate, patient intervention.

The aim of this chapter is to present innovation in TEL during and in response to COVID-19 and provide Torbay use cases that can inspire and potentially be replicated across other healthcare organisations. It presents an overview of existing TEL services at TSDFT, the process of TEL innovation adopted during COVID-19, examples of use cases developed to tackle COVID-19 challenges, and a discussion about sustainability and ongoing challenges for implementing and scaling up TEL services. Innovation in TEL for COVID-19 must be documented and evaluated, and use cases and clinical evidence must be developed so that TEL solutions can be made more inclusive, personalised and empowering for the learners (Guze, 2015). Critically reflecting upon and then sharing use cases can help in guiding the future of medical education (Goh and Sandars, 2020).

1.2. Existing TEL services at Torbay

TSDFT has a variety of digital tools and learning technologies such as Simulation (Sim) Labs, The Digital Futures Hub, The VR Lab, Hive Learning Management System (LMS) and in-house livestream TV and video recording studio. The purpose of our TEL programme is to support evolving education and training requirements of the hospital with a focus on the delivery of technical and non-technical skills training for staff and undergraduate students.

For example, prior to the pandemic, the simulation and Digital Futures teams worked together to deliver 360-degree VR simulations that incorporated high-fidelity computerised manikins and simulated environments, alongside role play by actors and clinical educators in order to meet curriculum delivery requirements. A particular area of emphasis has been on teaching first-person perspectives to medical students through patient-point-of-view recorded scenarios presented in VR. In addition, the Digital Futures Hub has also been supporting hospital teams to manage pain and anxiety in their patients through the loan of VR and AR headsets providing distraction interventions (with provision of guidance on best practices including hygiene and information governance).

However, throughout 2020, our team has expanded currently available TEL tools and services as a response to address the emerging COVID-19 challenges.

1.3. *Innovation of TEL through design thinking methodology*

Witnessing the worldwide surge in COVID-19 cases, TSDFT began preparing strategies and anticipating critical scenarios. A team of simulation experts, learning technologists and clinicians came together to brainstorm and develop solutions for the emerging challenges in the priority areas of supporting healthcare workers, medical students and patients. COVID-19 exerted pressures on the healthcare systems calling for unprecedented approaches towards rapid ideation and adoption. Pragmatism-led design thinking methodology enabled teams to expand and adapt existing TEL to best meet the end-user's requirements, in a short period of time.

Innovation within healthcare generally follows the path of recognition of problems, assessment of available resources and requirements, procurement, intervention assignment, evaluation, reiteration and reassignment of interventions. Additional time is then spent in ensuring the interventions are adopted on a larger scale. From start to finish, this process can take years before the new solutions become part of standard healthcare practice. However, the current pandemic is critical, difficult to predict and requires decisive actions.

Design thinking is a methodology often used within software development to solve complex problems in a pragmatic manner. As an innovation methodology, design thinking is slowly being integrated within healthcare innovation research (McLaughlin *et al.*, 2019). It requires input from a combination of a diverse multidisciplinary teams and end-users, as brainstorming together can help in 'rapid prototyping' (McLaughlin *et al.*, 2019). Pragmatic thinking greatly reduces the number of iterations required through the ideation, prototyping and testing phases. According to Dalsgaard (2014), John Dewey's pragmatic philosophy, which proposes that our understanding of the world is based on consequences and practice, is the scaffolding for design thinking (Dewey, 1938). Applying an experience-based approach over doctrines can be more efficient as it enables teams to recognise problems and arrive at solutions in a short timeframe (Schön, 1985). Another important aspect of design thinking is that iterations can be made at any point during the innovation process, using real-time inputs from end-users for whom the interventions are developed. End-users play the role of co-creators by offering inputs based on their personal experiences, which helps ensure that the solutions developed are practical and usable in real-world scenarios.

At TSDFT, the clinicians, educators and learning technologists worked together to deliver TEL solutions for COVID-19. Diverse and multidisciplinary teams made up of end-users and developers cut down the time required to research the gaps, generate ideas, develop designs, receive approvals and deliver quick implementation. The clinicians and educators were able to assist learning technologists by describing the problems and helping develop solutions that meet their individual COVID-19 requirements. Vitally, these conversations were not driven from a technology-first approach, but designed to focus on the human need at the centre of the challenge.

The design thinking model we used is the 'double diamond' process proposed by (British Council, 2020) made up of four phases as presented in Figure 1. The model is not linear as teams can go back and forth through the stages as required.

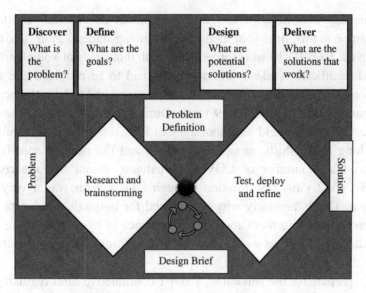

Figure 1. Design thinking double diamond (The British Design Council, 2020).

Using this double-diamond process, clinicians, educators and learning technologists at TSDFT actively engaged in strategising roles, leadership, task allocation and setting deadlines for individual projects. Ideas were implemented as soon as they were developed, and at the same time, the new developments underwent changes in order to improve usability.

2. Torbay Hospital's TEL Use Cases for COVID-19

2.1. *Priority: Healthcare workers*

2.1.1. *Challenge 1: Training of new staff/existing staff for unfamiliar roles*

COVID-19 has exerted exceptional pressures on hospitals around the world, which often operated at maximum capacity even during pre-COVID-19 times. During the early days of the pandemic, hospitals had to redeploy existing staff to COVID-19 wards due to staff shortages. In addition to this, final-year medical and nursing students graduated early to join the COVID-19 workforce, along with thousands of volunteers and retired healthcare workers. Most workers had to be retrained and reacquainted with healthcare environments and many had to be introduced to the management of COVID-19 work. During the early days of the pandemic, the entire world saw shortages in PPE supplies. This, combined with long tiring shifts, anxiety and stress and the need to care for an unprecedented number of COVID-19 patients, meant that the risk of SARS-CoV-2 virus transmission through human error was a very real concern. This is precisely why it is crucial for hospitals to educate staff and keep reminding them about the importance of hygiene and safe donning/doffing of PPE as well as provide any additional training required to make their work less stressful.

To prepare for the pandemic, TSDFT continued to offer regularly run training simulations. These could be accessed in person (in limited group numbers to ensure social distancing) or through HIVE LMS (online). Simulation scenarios included training of basic skills such as hygiene practices, patient communication, donning/doffing of PPE and turning a patient prone in order to support the treatment on a ventilator. Scenarios were filmed as 360-degree videos, offering first-person perspectives of COVID-19 wards and actual working environments. These simulations enabled staff to develop awareness of the hazards associated with high-risk areas and make errors in a consequence-free safe environment. This gave staff an opportunity to learn and become better prepared for work in COVID-19 wards.

2.1.2. *Challenge 2: Adapting and communication through PPE*

Effective communication is critical in healthcare, but especially in high-risk areas, such as the intensive care unit (ICU) or operating theatre. Failure to communicate critical information can lead to error with serious consequences for the patient. It is also vital that healthcare professionals communicate effectively with patients and their families. During the COVID-19 pandemic, healthcare teams are required to wear full PPE, which can make it impossible for people to read facial expressions. This is further compounded by the muffling of voices by the N95 masks. Shortages in PPE supplies and risk of virus transmission have meant that healthcare workers cannot keep donning and doffing PPE suits and masks.

TSDFT's Digital Futures team has produced a 6-min, 360-degree simulation video that gives the patients perspective of interacting with healthcare staff wearing PPE. This has been used for training healthcare workers in the critical skill of providing reassurance and effective, clear communication, while wearing PPE. Feedback gained from this virtual experience is being used to inform and improve simulation workshops for teaching effective team communication and affirming gestures.

2.1.3. *Challenge 3: Process mapping*

Torbay hospital has undergone significant layout changes as the ICU COVID-19 isolation wards had to be expanded. New and existing staff must be able to navigate these layouts and be able to direct COVID-19 and non-COVID-19 patients to the correct wards. Any errors could lead to potential cross-infection and outbreaks.

Digital Futures team captured a series of 360-degree videos of the hospital in order to support process mapping and virtual tours. These videos can be accessed through the HIVE LMS (online) or via VR headsets. Filmed from first-person perspective, these videos allow staff to quickly become acclimatised to their new workspace by mapping spaces virtually and allowing environments to be deconstructed with interactive information pop-ups and 'hot spots'.

2.1.4. *Challenge 4: Employee mental well-being*

The COVID-19 pandemic is unlike anything we have experienced before. Stressed healthcare workers are working around the clock in exceedingly difficult environments which are not only physically but also mentally exhausting. Open and transparent communication from senior leaders is important for connecting teams and maintaining morale during these truly isolating times. Video messages are recorded by executives using the in-house live TV studio to be streamed to TSDFT staff across all sites. At the outset of the pandemic, the NHS procured Microsoft (MS) Teams, which has been used to connect teams for virtual meetings as well as one-on-one or group debriefing. Mental health counselling is also available via MS Teams for employees.

Digital Futures partnered with Birmingham University's Human Interface Technologies (HIT) Team pre-COVID-19 to offer a therapeutic VR experience showing a David Attenborough-type nature experience. This VR experience showcases scenic mountain scenarios with Sir David Attenborough providing a breathing exercise and calming narration. In addition, a curated library of nature-based escapism experiences was also made available on VR. These experiences (paired with donated massage chairs) in a well-being space offered staff a well-deserved respite during shift breaks. Prior to COVID-19, we followed a strict hygiene protocol for cleaning headsets which was improved with the addition of UV cleaning boxes in order to meet COVID-19 requirements. The hygiene protocol we use has been signed off by TSDFT's Infection Control and has been used as a template for VR headsets nationally.

2.2. Priority: Healthcare students

2.2.1. Challenge 1: Healthcare student programmes

TSDFT hosts medical students from Plymouth and Exeter Universities, but due to the COVID-19 risks, students were not able to attend practical training or face-to-face classroom sessions. As face-to-face was no longer a viable option, clinical educators and facilitators began to run virtual classrooms through MS Teams. Additional educational material related to practical sessions is available on the Trusts Vimeo channel and LMS. The comments sections on these videos are active with interaction between students and educators. The studio space was also used to create teaching materials that captured material usually delivered face-to-face and converted it to remote on-demand video content.

2.3. Priority: Patients

2.3.1. Challenge 1: COVID-19 patient experience

TSDFT's TEL programme was expanded to aid COVID-19 patients and improve their quality of care. Being alone in isolation, away from family, not knowing whether one is going to get better and see their loved ones again is a very fearful experience. Although some patients may have their phones with them, many don't or are too unwell to use them without assistance. Through the TEL programme, we offer iPads with splash guards and rugged cases, to the patients. The iPads come loaded with the Lifelines app which enables patients in ICU and their families to have virtual visits. There is also an email account that family and friends can write to if their loved one is in ICU that is monitored frequently.

2.3.2. Challenge 2: Non-COVID-19 patient experience

Priority access to healthcare has meant that only patients requiring critical care are able to get appointments. Patients with manageable symptoms are asked to stay home and safe, and avoid unnecessary exposure to the virus. These patients can connect to healthcare professionals with the nationally procured Attend Anywhere telehealth application. Attend Anywhere lets patients connect with clinicians or nurses over video at assigned time slots. This is reassuring for patients and ensures that they can continue to receive the care they require during the pandemic.

Figures 2, 3 and 4 present a visualisation of the use cases described above.

3. Discussion

The COVID-19 pandemic has presented global healthcare with unprecedented challenges. However, it has also offered opportunities for healthcare teams to collaborate on the implementation of innovation at a significantly accelerated pace. There are several factors that have enabled TSDFT to incorporate design thinking methodology and innovate TEL solutions to meet the COVID-19 challenges. In this section, we also

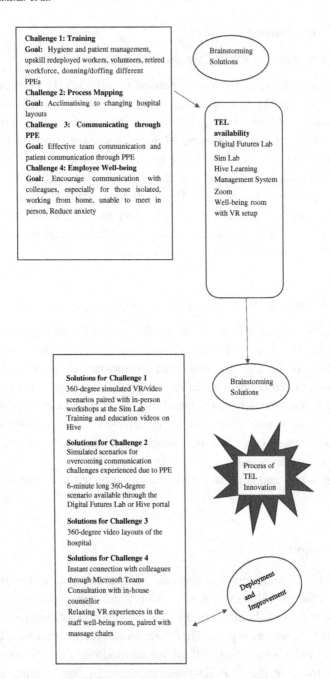

Challenge 1: Training
Goal: Hygiene and patient management, upskill redeployed workers, volunteers, retired workforce, donning/doffing different PPEs
Challenge 2: Process Mapping
Goal: Acclimatising to changing hospital layouts
Challenge 3: Communicating through PPE
Goal: Effective team communication and patient communication through PPE
Challenge 4: Employee Well-being
Goal: Encourage communication with colleagues, especially for those isolated, working from home, unable to meet in person, Reduce anxiety

Brainstorming Solutions

TEL availability
Digital Futures Lab
Sim Lab
Hive Learning Management System
Zoom
Well-being room with VR setup

Solutions for Challenge 1
360-degree simulated VR/video scenarios paired with in-person workshops at the Sim Lab
Training and education videos on Hive

Solutions for Challenge 2
Simulated scenarios for overcoming communication challenges experienced due to PPE

6-minute long 360-degree scenario available through the Digital Futures Lab or Hive portal

Solutions for Challenge 3
360-degree video layouts of the hospital

Solutions for Challenge 4
Instant connection with colleagues through Microsoft Teams
Consultation with in-house counsellor
Relaxing VR experiences in the staff well-being room, paired with massage chairs

Brainstorming Solutions

Process of TEL Innovation

Deployment and Improvement

Figure 2.   TEL innovation in healthcare workers domain.

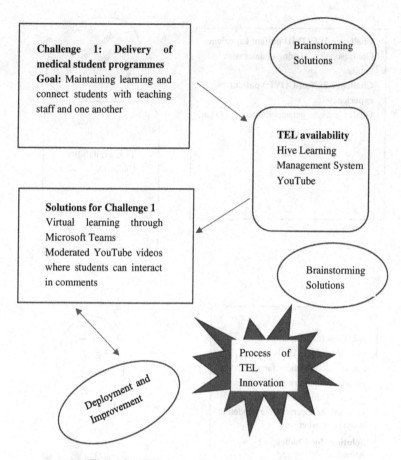

Figure 3. TEL innovation in students domain.

consider the sustainability of these innovations and explore future opportunities.

3.1. *Team approach*

Gaining empathetic insights into the experience of clinicians, students and patients has allowed TSDFT to develop a supportive network wherein every stakeholder is able to contribute through their experience and skills. Teamwork and open communication continue to be the backbone of innovative development at Torbay.

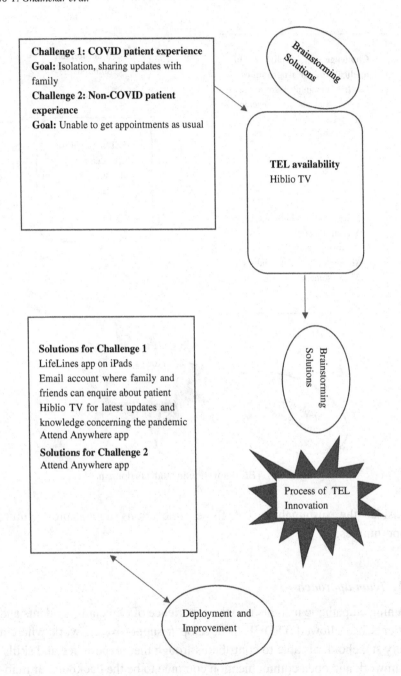

Figure 4.   TEL innovation in patients domain.

3.2. *Prior experience and TEL availability*

TSDFT has an advantage in immersive learning technologies implementation. For the past five years, our hospital has been involved in VR research and practice through being the first HEE-funded NHS VR Lab. Torbay has access to a variety of VR headsets (Oculus Quest, Oculus Go, HTC Vive, Pico Neo 3) and 360-degree cameras, technicians, researchers and clinicians who are experienced at debriefing immersive simulation workshops. We have also facilitated other hospitals within our network to set up their own VR programmes.

3.3. *Sustainability of interventions*

Ensuring long-term sustainability of the interventions developed will be key towards transforming future practice. This will be underpinned by developing an evidence base for impact through undertaking TEL-based research alongside service quality improvement evaluations. We are specifically interested in studying the role of simulations in PPE training, mental health and the transformations that can be achieved within medical education. It is important to establish empirical data on feasibility and acceptability in order to support sustained spread and adoption. Our current situation does not afford us the time required to conduct these evaluations; however, we plan on studying the effect of the changes we have implemented when resources allow.

3.4. *Future delivery*

The solutions we have developed aim to address temporary problems created by the pandemic, but we are anticipating certain long-term challenges, too.

3.4.1. *Medical education and training*

The transformative effects of COVID-19 on education can be witnessed globally. Traditional didactic sessions presented in classrooms have moved online. As students get used to the 'new normal', medical students will continue to face challenges as their exposure to practical, clinical experience will be restricted. Although tele-education can meet certain requirements, it cannot provide authentic patient experiences (Rose, 2020) and critical clinical skills cannot develop if students do not experience patient engagement. Mian and Khan (2020) recommend providing students with access through patient-held tablets that can be cleaned using infection control protocols. TSDFT has access to iPads with splash guards that could be used to provide students with direct access to COVID-19 patients.

Johnson and Blitzer (2020) suggest interactions with real and virtual patients can help fill face-to-face training gaps. The authors also suggest partnering with video gaming companies to create authentic virtual clinical experiences that meet the accredited competency requirements. Torbay's partnership with South Devon College (SDC), UK, (who have game design students) will be leveraged to create such scenarios if required by the educators. Another issue that educators may face is students may get so familiar with virtual learning (and its convenience) that they will not return to classroom settings once the pandemic is under control. However, this may not be a challenge, but an opportunity to transform medical education for the better. If virtual learning can engage students effectively, then this could become the 'new normal'. As Rose (2020) recommends, students and clinical educators must collaborate and contribute towards this change in practice if it is to truly meet needs and become embedded.

3.4.2. *Healthcare workers' training*

TEL simulations can virtually replicate real work situations, highlight key issues such as team communication and create a safe environment for healthcare workers to train. The feedback received from the users can assist in improving the simulations and through this, clinical practice. However, simulations cannot completely substitute for real clinical environments and, therefore, where appropriate and under careful considerations, we continue to run *in-situ* participant-based simulations using social distancing. Healthcare workers, specifically volunteers who may not have clinical experience, may behave completely different within real settings. Therefore, it is important to continue some level of face-to-face training.

3.4.3. *Healthcare workers' physical and mental health*

The hospital will be providing more resources to help staff in dealing with returning to work, stress, anxiety, depression and post-traumatic stress disorder (PTSD). We are working on expanding simulations in meditation and breathing exercises. Collaboration with clinical psychology, occupational health and workforce development teams will help us in developing simulations to support specific mental health conditions.

3.4.4. *Sustainability of Digital Futures*

The Digital Futures Hub will be used to support the workforce in acquiring the digital skills and competencies required in order for our staff to feel digital 'ready'. This will be achieved through running a programme of workshops, technology 'deep dives', and supported digital drop-in clinics as well as continuing our co-design workshops. Additionally, working alongside both industry and academic partners, Digital Futures will aim to support digital research and QI projects, which will be funded through our ability to seek grants and trailblaze projects in our speciality XR technology space.

Specifically, Digital Futures will look to support the skills gap, caused by COVID-19 with our postgraduate trainees, by providing an understanding of the current and emerging digital technologies landscape. This will influence future careers by providing a theoretical and hands-on understanding of digital tools in delivering healthcare, education and research. This work is mapped as a response to findings and recommendations in the HEE Topol Review, 2019.

3.5. *Hygiene of TEL devices*

A separate and important piece of learning is how to adapt TEL solutions to be practically implemented in the COVID-19 world. The SARS-CoV-2 virus can survive on surfaces and may be transmitted through contact with infected surfaces. At Torbay, any devices used by multiple people are cleaned and disinfected thoroughly by trained TEL staff. Specifically, the cleaning of VR headsets is critical as even with the users wearing disposable face masks, viral transmission can occur if disinfection and hygiene practices are not followed. Based on guidelines developed with the Infection Control at Torbay hospital, devices are cleaned using medical-grade cleaning wipes and a UV cleaning box. Disposable face masks that cover all areas of the headset which touch the user's face are also used as additional protection against transmission of infection. Employees responsible for delivering simulations have all been trained in hygienic handling of the devices.

4. Conclusion

The aim of presenting our TEL use cases for addressing the COVID-19 challenges is to encourage other healthcare providers to start a discussion and potentially working towards developing their own use cases. Through a human-centric approach driven by empathy, pragmatism and openness towards the possibilities of technology, most healthcare organisations can build structures to support their staff, students and patients during these difficult times. As documented by (Li *et al.*, 2020), TEL has played a key role in helping Chinese healthcare workers deal with COVID-19. We are hoping to replicate similar success at TSDFT using the TEL modalities at our disposal.

We aim to create additional simulation scenarios specifically created for the education and training of individuals and teams. We will produce additional 360-degree content to support healthcare workers and incorporate AR for tele-education. As COVID-19 trends change, hospital priorities will shift. We plan on modelling TEL to meet transforming needs. Safety of health personnel is an essential global concern (Huh, 2020) and our focus remains on ensuring mental and physical well-being of our staff. We will continue to investigate how virtual learning can be integrated into programmes as a substitute for classroom teaching and real-life patient experiences, without compromising on the acquisition of key skills.

Exploring how technology can be used to connect patients and their families (especially those in COVID-19 isolation wards) will remain a priority as we regard that the hospital's role is to ensure not only the physical but also the mental well-being of its community.

The inspiration for this chapter is derived from Li *et al.*'s (2020) explanation that learning technologies and immersive simulations are resource-consuming. The digital teams at TSDFT already have in-house video/film and VR production abilities, along with the latest VR headsets, and TEL staff are trained in VR hygiene. Rapid innovation, expansion and adaptation of the COVID-19 TEL solutions were straightforward as TSDFT has experience of developing and implementing learning technologies. But, we also believe these successes are replicable. More importantly, the benefits of integrating learning technologies outweigh the investment in the resources required. With the presentation of the different TEL developments at TSDFT, we hope to educate and inspire other healthcare providers around the world to transform their practices. Our 'new normal' must be developed in a manner where we are still able to salvage and retain human connection through one of the most impactful resources available — technology.

References

Baxendale, B. (2017) Simulation and technology enhanced learning: Future implications for healthcare education and practice. *BMJ Simulation and Technology Enhanced Learning*, 3(Suppl 3). doi: 10.1136/bmjstel-2017-demec.edit.

Council, D. (2020) Eleven lessons: Managing design in eleven global brands — A study of the design process. Available at: https://www.designcouncil.org.uk/fileadmin/uploads/dc/Documents/ElevenLessons_Design_Council%2520%25282%2529.pdf.

Dalsgaard, P. (2014) Pragmatism and design thinking. *International Journal of Design*, 8(1), 143–155.

Dewey, J. (1938) *Experience and Education*. McMillan Company, New York.

Goh, P.-S. and Sandars, J. (2020) A vision of the use of technology in medical education after the COVID-19 pandemic. *MedEdPublish* (Preprint).

Grimwood, T. and Snell, L. (2020) The use of technology in healthcare education: A literature review. *MedEdPublish*, 9. doi: 10.15694/mep.2020.000137.1.

Guze, P. A. (2015) Using technology to meet the challenges of medical education. *Transactions of the American Clinical and Climatological Association*, 126, 260–270.

Huh, S. (2020) How to train health personnel to protect themselves from SARS-CoV-2 (novel coronavirus) infection when caring for a patient or suspected case. Department of Parasitology and Institute of Medical Education, College of Medicine, College of Medicine, Hallym University, Chuncheon, Korea (Preprint). Available at: http://jeehp.org/DOIx.php?id=10.3352/jeehp.2020.17.10.

Johnson, W. R. and Blitzer, D. (2020) Residents' perspectives on graduate medical education during the COVID-19 pandemic and beyond. *MedEdPublish*, 9(1). doi: 10.15694/mep.2020.000077.1.

Li, L., *et al.* (2020) Preparing and responding to 2019 novel coronavirus with simulation and technology-enhanced learning for healthcare professionals: Challenges and opportunities in China. *BMJ Simulation and Technology Enhanced Learning*. doi: 10.1136/bmjstel-2020-000609.

Madani, A., *et al.* (2017) Evaluating the role of simulation in healthcare innovation: Recommendations of the Simnovate Medical Technologies Domain Group. *BMJ Simulation and Technology Enhanced Learning*, 3(Suppl 1). doi: 10.1136/bmjstel-2016-000178.

McLaughlin, J. E., Wolcott, M. D., Hubbard, D., Umstead, K. & Rider, T. R. (2019) A qualitative review of the design thinking framework in health professions education. *BMC Medical Education*, 19(98). Available at: https://bmcmededuc.biomedcentral.com/articles/10.1186/s12909-019-1528-8.

Mian, A. and Khan, S. (2020) Medical education during pandemics: A UK perspective. *BMC Medicine*, 18(1), 100. doi: 10.1186/s12916-020-01577-y.

Osborne, F., *et al.* (2021) Using medical reality television as a technology-enhanced learning strategy to provide authentic patient care experiences during clinical placements: A case study research investigation. *BMC Medical Education*, 21(1), 15. doi: 10.1186/s12909-020-02432-7.

Rose, S. (2020) Medical student education in the time of COVID-19. *JAMA* (Preprint). doi: 10.1001/jama.2020.5227.

https://doi.org/10.1142/9781800614192_0007

Chapter 7

VR in Adult Acute Pain Management — An Exploration into the Existing Academic Literature

Salman Heydari Khajehpour*,‡, Mona Seyed Esfahani†,§, and Danylo Yershov*,¶

University Hospitals Dorset NHS Foundation Trust, Bournemouth, UK

†*Bournemouth University, Bournemouth, UK*

‡*Salman.HeydariKhajehpour@uhd.nhs.uk*
§*mseyedesfahani@bournemouth.ac.uk*
¶*danylo.yershov@nhs.net*

Health organisations around the world are constantly seeking tools and methods to manage patients' pain more effectively. This has been in the forefront of pain research for decades. Methods such as hypnosis, meditation and relaxation techniques alongside technological tools such as the use of video, audio and gaming are applied and investigated. With the advancement of technology, new tools such as Virtual Reality (VR) are used more and proved to be effective. However, the effectiveness of VR seems to be highly dependent on context, patients, measurements and applications. This chapter looks into the application of VR in Acute Pain management, common areas where it is used in and how it is evaluated. The chapter concludes by providing recommendations for enhancing the use of VR in the management of acute pain and offering insights into what to expect in the future.

1. Introduction

Pain is an unavoidable side effect of medical procedures and health problems. Everyday, almost 10 million people in UK alone suffer from pain (British Pain Society). Managing pain is costly. British Pain Society reported an estimated £5 million per year is spent on managing back pain alone. The traditional and most common pathway to pain management is pharmaceutical, however, this is changing. The shift is due to various side effects and overdependency to pain medications, which have resulted in an increase in mortality related to drug abuse. In recent years, there has been a global effort to provide non-pharmaceutical pain management techniques and many technological innovations have been trialled and tested as solutions. However, the search for an effective non-pharmaceutical alternative is still going on.

Innovation is the driving factor in the success of healthcare industry. National Health Services (NHS) England has addressed the importance of innovation as a tool that 'help(s) to prevent diseases, speed up diagnosis, improve safety and efficiency of services and increase patient participation in decision making, self-management and research. This will lead to better health outcomes and a more sustainable NHS' (Seyed Esfahani *et al.*, 2022, p. 1). One particular innovative technology receiving a lot of attention in the UK is Virtual Reality (VR). VR was introduced in the 1990s and soon after became commercially available and more accessible. VR is one of the advanced technologies being tested in pain management which is growing rapidly and is expected to be worth over $200 billion by 2024 (Statista, 2022). This chapter looks into the effect of VR in pain management, the common areas of use and how VR has been evaluated. To understand the advancement of VR technology in pain management, the concept of pain is going to be explored and VR technology is going to be looked at in more detail.

1.1. *Pain*

The International Association for the Study of Pain (IASP) defines pain as 'An unpleasant sensory and emotional experience associated with, or resembling that associated with, actual or potential tissue damage' (IASP, 2020). This definition is the most holistic concept of pain. They also published six keynotes and etymologies:

- 'Pain is always a personal experience that is influenced to varying degrees by biological, psychological and social factors.
- Pain and nociception are different phenomena. Pain cannot be inferred solely from activity in sensory neurons.
- Through their life experiences, individuals learn the concept of pain.
- A person's report of an experience as pain should be respected.
- Although pain usually serves an adaptive role, it may have adverse effects on function and social and psychological well-being' (IASP, 2020).

Pain is commonly described through verbal communication, however, this is not the only way pain experience is communicated. The absence of communication does not negate the possibility that an individual is experiencing pain.

Pain inflicted during surgery or by an injury, such as burn, is transmitted by way of sensory information from the peripheries via primary sensory neurones to the central nervous system (CNS). The body of all sensory neurons is located in the dorsal root ganglion. The peripheral nerve fibres are either large myelinated (A-alpha or A-beta), small myelinated (A-delta or B) or unmyelinated (C). Pain is transmitted through the small myelinated and unmyelinated sensory fibres. The sensory nerve endings are named 'peripheral nociceptor terminal'. These terminals have receptors and ion channels for inflammatory mediators produced by tissue injury and inflammation. The inflammatory mediators such as prostaglandins, bradykinin, cytokines, adenosine triphosphate (ATP), etc. activate intracellular signalling pathways, which increases the sensitivity of the peripheral nociceptor terminal to sensory stimuli. This process is named 'peripheral sensitisation' and can cause spontaneous pain.

Gate Control Theory (GCT) is proposed by Melzack and Wall (1965), explaining how pain is experienced. This theory suggests that the spinal cord contains a neurological 'gate' whereby the pain signals are transmitted to the brain. These gates either block pain signals, therefore decreasing pain perception and suffering, or allow them to continue, which means increasing pain perception. There are factors aggravating pain, such as focusing on pain and anxiety, and other factors decreasing pain by closing the gate and lessening the suffering, such as distraction and medication (Melzack and Wall, 1965). Based on this theory, methods that can create distraction or stress relief environment can reduce the pain and be effective in patient's pain management.

1.2. *Acute pain*

Acute pain is defined as pain lasting less than 12 weeks. (The British Pain Society), such as post-operative pain, which is short-lived and well controlled by multimodal analgesia. Nevertheless, there are a small number of patients whose pain is poorly controlled and who continue to suffer for prolonged periods of time, with a small number of them developing chronic pain. Chronic pain can be the result of an injury (e.g. trauma, surgery) or diseases (e.g. diabetes, cancer) or of an unknown origin (e.g. fibromyalgia) (Jensen *et al.*, 2011). This study focuses on acute pain. It is vital to choose the right therapy or combination of therapies early in the path of the acute pain to improve patient experience and quality of life, decrease length of stay in hospital and prevent chronicity. It is clear that prolonged pain is associated with decreased function and movement and could cause complications, disability and significant suffering and distress. Finally, this all translates into more cost for the NHS, which determines the importance of identifying pain management tools and techniques including pharmaceutical and non-pharmaceutical means to improve acute pain and prevent chronicity.

1.3. *Pharmacological therapy*

Pharmacological therapy is currently the main source of any pain control in primary and secondary care. According to the World Health Organization (WHO) ladder of pain, analgesia is started with non-opiate analgesic (e.g. paracetamol, non-steroidal anti-inflammatory) on a regular basis and then escalated to mild or moderate opiates (e.g. codeine, tramadol) and finally strong opiates (e.g. morphine, oxycodone) to control severe pain. However, these steps are bypassed in acute severe pain by a combination of multimodal analgesia used from the outset or prescription of strong opiates. Within the ladder, additional drugs like adjuvants may be used that include antidepressants (e.g. amitriptyline), anticonvulsants (e.g. gabapentin), corticosteroids (e.g. dexamethasone) and anxiolytics (e.g. diazepam).

1.4. *Non-pharmacological*

Non-pharmacologic alternative pain therapies have been used as a pathway to pain management for a long time, some rooted back to hundred years. Currently, alternative medicine is most frequently used and serves as an effective adjunctive therapy to treat chronic pain and typically musculoskeletal subtype. In some instances, such as in migraine, it helps to decrease and prevent the number of acute attacks.

Some examples of alternative therapies are acupuncture, Tai Chi, osteopathic manipulation and chiropractic care. Acupuncture, traditionally a Chinese practice, is becoming more popular across the world as a way to relieve pain. However, there is very little use of these methods in acute pain in the Western world. Other non-pharmaceutical alternatives have been explored by medical experts for years, in particular cognitive therapy (Meldrum, 2003), distraction and Relaxation techniques (e.g. Johnson, 2005; Ahmadpour *et al.*, 2019).

Programmes such as the Pain Management Programme (PMP) have explored non-pharmaceutical options and psychology-based rehabilitative treatment for people with chronic pain that has remained unresolved by other treatments currently available (The British Pain Society). The aim of the PMP is to improve pain sufferers' quality of life and not necessarily their level of pain and is based on techniques to learn about and manage pain, such as relaxation and exercise (NHS UK). Traditional technologies such as watching movies (Cohen *et al.*, 1999), listening to music (Fowler-Kerry and Lander, 1987), counting objects in the room (Zeltzer *et al.*, 1991) and having nonmedical conversations (Blount *et al.*, 1994) are used as a means of distraction (Wismeijer and Vingerhoets, 2005). Later development of technology resulted in the emergence of advanced tools such as VR as an emerging and effective non-pharmaceutical treatment for pain relief (Ding *et al.*, 2020).

2. Virtual Reality

The virtual world is used to immerse the patient in a 3D environment and mimic real sensory experience (Ahn, 2011; Ahn *et al.*, 2016). This increases their level of presence in the virtual world and takes their focus away from the pain. Advances in the VR software and hardware allow accurate tracking of users' bodies, thereby improving user immersion (Handa *et al.*, 2012). VR technology is advancing and new software with more realistic environments, which allow better user engagement and interaction, are introduced to the marketplace frequently. Advanced headsets have proven to be more comfortable and offer more accessible and interactive features. In some areas, the use of VR has been established and proven to be effective, such as rehabilitation (Hoffman, 2004; North *et al.*, 1997; Massetti *et al.*, 2018), treatment of eating disorders (Ferrer-Garcia *et al.*, 2013), phobia, post-traumatic stress disorder (PTSD) (Hoffman, 2004), mental disorders (Maples-Keller *et al.*, 2017) and chemical abuse (Hoe-Blanchet *et al.*, 2014), burn (Soltani *et al.* 2018), orthopaedics (Li *et al.*, 2018) and episiotomy (Jahanishoorab *et al.*, 2015). However, this is not always the case (e.g. Jin *et al.*, 2018; Ding *et al.*, 2019; Yang *et al.*, 2019).

The success of VR is attributed to its ability to transfer users to an engaging and interactive environment, making patients feel like they are a part of the virtual environment (VE) (Matheve *et al.*, 2020). Patients involved in this interactive and immersive environment find their attention diverted from pain (Li *et al.*, 2017). However, the use of VR as a non-pharmaceutical intervention has not always yielded a positive result. The reasons behind the mixed findings are not definitively determined. However, studies have shed light on several factors that contribute to these variations, including the diverse application of virtual reality (VR), variations in settings, differences among patients, environmental factors, and methodological approaches. In order to explore the limitation, the application of VR needs to be explained.

2.1. *VR as passive and active distraction*

VR is vastly used as a distraction or relaxation intervention (e.g. Johnson, 2005) to distract individuals from the pain they are experiencing or to transmit individuals into a relaxed and calming environment (i.e. Dascal *et al.*, 2017). Distraction means shifting or moving one's attention away from the pain to another cortex stimulus. It does not mean that the pain is no longer there. One of the objectives is to limit the amount of time you spend worrying about or being afraid of pain. Based on the assumption that 'pain perception has a large psychological component in that the amount of attention directed to the noxious stimuli modulated the perceived pain' (Wismeijer and Vingerhoets, 2005, p. 268), the distraction techniques consume suffers' limited attention capacity and result in the removal of attention away from pain stimuli. It is argued that the idea of the distraction technique is based on the consumption of an optimum amount of attention that involves numerous sensory modalities (audio, video, kinesthetics) (Slifer, 2002). Audiovisual (A/V) techniques such as watching movies and listening to music were advanced and included multiple sensory stimuli presented in a 2D or 3D environment and were initially named A/V distraction, VR or A/V eyeglass system (Wismeijer and Vingerhoets, 2005).

VR distraction (VRD) is defined as 'a human–computer interface that enables the user to interact dynamically with the computer-generated environment' (Wismeijer *et al.*, 2005, p. 268), aiming to help with patient behaviour management. This is also called active distraction, as individuals are actively involved in performing a task, such as shooting a target. The intervention blocks out the 'external stimuli that may provoke a negative attitude' (Felemban *et al.*, 2021, p. 2). Using VR as a distraction tool has proved effective in pain management within various contexts such as burn (e.g. Sharar *et al.*, 2007), dentistry (e.g. Felemban *et al.*, 2021), gynaecology (e.g. Jahanshoorab *et al.*, 2015), urology (e.g. Walker *et al.*, 2014) and colorectal (e.g. Ding *et al.*, 2019).

Relaxation, or passive distraction, averts individuals' attention from the pain using inactive content, such as relaxation (Inan and Inal, 2019). When VR is used as a relaxation tool, the intervention contains a programme that creates a calming environment, such as images of a beach or forest. This method is used in various contexts, e.g. burn (e.g. Konstantatos *et al.*, 2009), orthopaedic surgery (e.g. Faruki *et al.*, 2019), gynaecology (e.g. Deo *et al.*, 2021) and obstetrics (e.g. Frey *et al.*, 2019). Nowadays, high-tech headsets offer high-resolution interactive environments and create a more realistic experience for users. Distraction is proved effective in some areas such as postoperative pain to not only reduce pain by distracting the sufferer from the pain, but also by alleviating negative emotions such as fear and anxiety that can result in more brain activity in the emotion-related medical pain system (Jerdan *et al.*, 2018; Ding *et al.*, 2020).

Virtual reality is used in various contexts and proved effective and impactful. The technology is used in the management of acute and chronic pain, however, this study only explores the research around acute pain on adult participants. Some areas have benefited from the technology longer than others. This can be attributed to the higher demand and desperation of pain sufferers, such as those with burns, or to the greater flexibility in applying VR intervention due to setting management, as seen in dentistry. VR experiments are conducted with both healthy participants and patients. Using healthy participants allows the researcher to be more flexible with the research design, whereas using patients limits the design, acknowledging patients' conditions, prioritising their treatment, safety and comfort. From examining the literature, it is also evident that the effectiveness of VR is evaluated differently, and depending on the setting, other factors are considered important and have an impact on the final assessment of the effectiveness of VR intervention. A literature search was done on VR for pain management across 4 databases: Pubmed, Medline, Embase and Cinahl. 144 non-duplicated studies were found. Out of those 144 studies, 8 studies involved paediatric population, 16 studies involved chronic pain and 41 studies were non-acute pain related. One study was found to not involve any data when extracted, so it was removed. This brought down the number of relevant articles of VR in acute pain management to 78. All of these articles have used VR to aid with identifying acute pain symptoms experienced while undergoing a procedure.

Based on the exploration of literature, the application of technology alongside measurement, context and research design is examined and explained further (Figure 1).

3. Virtual Reality Measurement

Studies looking into examining the suitability and applicability of VR as a non-pharmaceutical intervention in the area of pain management looked mainly into evaluating users' pain and discomfort level. The level of pain is measured using different scales. Numerical rating scale (NRS) is an analogue pain scale usually having the range of 1–10, 0–10 or 0–100, which indicates the pain intensity. 1 or 0 being 'no pain at all' and the

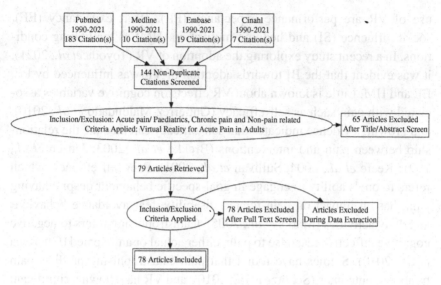

Figure 1.   Literature search diagram.

upper limit represents 'unbearable pain'. This scale is one of the most common scales used in pain evaluation followed by the visual analogue scale (VAS). VAS contains a horizontal line representing a continuing range of values. VAS has proved to be easy to use, valid and reliable (Gloth 3rd *et al.*, 2001; Scott and Huskisson, 1976). If any descriptive information such as mild or severe is added, then the scale is named graphic rating scale (GRS). Verbal rating scale (VRS) is not used as commonly. This scale refers to when users are asked to select an adjective that describes their level of pain. Some studies included cognitive, affective and sensory pain measurement scales. Cognitive refers to 'time spent thinking about pain', affective, to the level of unpleasantness perceived and sensory, to the intensity level of the pain.

Within the literature, there have always been discussions on correlations and moderating effect of other factors such as behavioural, cognitive and personality traits. For example, if an individual attributes the pain to a greater threat to their health, they may rate higher on affective pain dimension (Taenzer *et al.*, 1986; Wade *et al.*, 1990). According to a modified UTAUT, factors influencing behavioural intention (BI) towards the use of VR. are performance expectancy (PE), effort expectancy (EE), social influence (SI) and hedonic motivation (HM) as facilitating conditions. In a recent study exploring the adoption of VR (Toyoda *et al.*, 2021), it was evident that the BI towards adoption of VR was influenced by PE, EE and HM. Little is known about VR effects on cognitive variables associated with pain such as self-efficacy (Gutierrez-Maldndado *et al.*, 2010), and growing evidence indicates that self-efficacy can mediate the relationship between pain and interventions (Brekke *et al.*, 2003; Jensen *et al.*, 1991; Keefe *et al.*, 2004; Sullivan *et al.*, 2001). Pain self-efficacy, which refers to one's ability to engage in goal-specific behaviour despite having pain, has an impact on pain-related disability, fear avoidance behaviour and daily activities (Marks *et al.*, 2005). Catastrophising refers to negative cognitive–affective response to pain, either actual or anticipated (Quartana *et al.*, 2010). Studies have found that pain catastrophising predicts pain treatment outcomes (Schütze *et al.*, 2010), and VR has shown a significant effect on reducing pain catastrophising and increasing pain self-efficacy (e.g. Asghari Moghaddam, 2014; Sharifpour *et al.*, 2020).

Despite the importance of above-mentioned factors, pain self-efficacy, pain catastrophising and pain sensitivity are being included in a limited number of papers. Other behavioural factors identified in technology acceptance frameworks are rarely measured in clinical VR studies. This needs to be addressed in future research, as the context of VR application in pain management is truly an interdisciplinary area. Hence, considering behavioural factors impacting the acceptance of VR as a technology, such as self-expectancy and motivation, alongside pain-related factors with the same effect, such as self-efficacy and catastrophising, will enhance the validity and accuracy of the findings and broadens scholar's understanding of pain intervention outcomes.

3.1. *Evaluation of immersion in the VR environment*

VR is being used as an effective non-pharmaceutical intervention for pain management. Individuals either wear a headset or experience the virtual world via a screen. Users are then exposed to a content and are immersed in a VE. In the communication literature, VR has been defined as 'a real or simulated environment in which a perceiver experiences telepresence'

(Steuer, 1992, p. 7). Telepresence is the sense of being in the environment, in this case, the VE (Klein, 2003). Telepresence is enabled via user control (interactivity) and vividness (Steuer, 1992) which also applies in VR environments, as the perceptual VR experience can be measured via users' perceived interactivity and immersion (Bhatt, 2004). Interactivity is defined by its speed, range and significance, whereas immersion is deliberated through the breadth of immersion (i.e. the sum of sensory organs that are influenced by the VR) and depth of immersion (i.e. the degree of resolution) (Seyed Esfahani, 2016). Immersion refers to 'the feeling of being deeply engaged in a virtual world as if it were the real one' (Ragusa and Bochenek, 2001, cited in Bhatt, 2004, p. 5). Presence is added as a third characteristic of VR which relates to 'the subjective experience of being in one place or environment, even when one is physically in another' (Witmer and Singer, 1998, p. 225).

Presence is rarely included in VR and pain management studies. However, there is a strong body of literature supporting a positive correlation between perceived presence and VR acceptance (e.g. Plotzky *et al.*, 2021; Shin, Biocca and Choo, 2013), user engagement, positive experience and fun (e.g. Sra *et al.*, 2018). Gutierrez-Maldonado *et al.* (2010) have referred to sense of presence as the illusion of 'being there' in a virtual world, so that participants evoke the same reactions and emotions as in a real-world situation. Within the clinical context, presence, in particular spatial presence, is included in a few of the studies, and the effect of perceived presence is being explored. For example, Sharar *et al.* (2007), found out a correlation between sense of presence and the age of participants — the younger the users, the higher the level of perceived presence. Hodges *et al.* (1994) identified while treating psychological disorders that one of the key features of VR is the sense of presence, which is used to describe the illusion of 'being there'. This is explained as the property that results in the VR environment evoking the same reactions and emotions that are experienced in a non-VR environment (Hodges *et al.*, 1994). A high level of presence is associated with increased response to exposure therapy and a better outcome (Mitrousia and Giotakos, 2016). Also, the more the patient feels the presence, the more they believe in the illusion created in the VE, which can increase the effectiveness of VR treatment (Donegan *et al.*, 2020).

Discussion around presence also involves users' level of engagement and participation. Gutierrez-Maldonado *et al.* (2010) explain if patients can't involve themselves in a virtual world, they can't experience similar emotions and the 'habituation and extinction' process won't happen (p. 79). They further explain that presence is measured with three factors: sense of physical space, engagement/involvement and ecological validity/realism. Some academics believe that presence and involvement must be separated, one can be present but not involved and vice versa. Interestingly, this study indicated that involvement does not correlate with any of the pain measures and concluded that involvement might not be necessarily a dimension of presence.

4. Virtual Reality Context

VR application in pain management has been researched in different settings. Experiments in laboratory-based studies on healthy volunteers show benefits of VR in pain management. Clinical research reached similar conclusions in multiple specialities. VR has a great potential to be adopted in multiple branches of medicine as a tool to improve pain management. Laboratory-based research paved the way for employing VR in clinical practice. Multiple studies were conducted on healthy adult volunteers to investigate the impact of VR on pain perception. One of the main factors to be considered in these studies was identifying pain stimuli suitable for healthy adult participants. The stimuli need to be stimulating enough to create sufficient level of pain but not too painful. Also, participants' different pain thresholds need to be taken into account. However, only a few studies measured participants' pain thresholds before the experiment by asking participants to rate the pain induced by the stimuli and used the information to adjust the pain stimuli during the experiment. For example, Weeth *et al.* (2017) adjusted the amperage of the electrical stimuli based on participants' pain thresholds. As for stimuli, in case of healthy adult participants, electrical stimuli were used commonly. Other studies such as Magora *et al.* (2006) used a tourniquet to be inflated to the point the participants experience pain. Enea *et al.* (2014) used finger pressure pain, and thermal stimuli (hot or cold) are also used by some scholars (e.g. Hoffman, 2004; Loreto-Quijada *et al.*, 2014).

4.1. *VR's impact on pain perception — healthy participants*

Recruiting healthy participants results in more freedom in designing the study, hence the popularity of this sampling choice. Weeth *et al.* (2017), e.g. looked into the influence of a 'visually manipulated appearance of a virtual arm' on pain perception. The study aimed to investigate the reduction of perceived pain when participants were exposed to an image that visually induces the feeling of protection. The influence on pain perception was explored in a study of 32 participants (18–46 years). Volunteers used a head-mounted device (HMD) and software displaying a virtual arm in three states: uncovered (image of an arm with no clothes), neutral (image of an arm covered with a sleeve) and armoured (image of an arm with an iron armour). The naked unprotected arm represented an 'unprotected' state, the sleeve-covered arm represented the 'neutral' state and armoured arm represented the 'protected' state. Participants received electrical stimuli and compared their pain perception in the three states using a numeric pain score (0–100). Interestingly, subjects with virtual arm protection had a decreased perception of electrical stimuli.

Lier *et al.* (2020) studied the effect of VR on evoked potentials (EPs) (electrical response from a stimulation of a nerve) following painful electrical stimuli and subjective pain with the help of 30 healthy adult volunteers (18 and over). EPs are 'voltage changes in the electroencephalography (EEG) that occur within a specified time after a stimulus' (Lier *et al.*, 2020, p. 2). Three VR conditions were compared: passive VR (i.e. no interaction possible with the virtual world), active VR (interactive VE) and no VR (black screen). In the passive VR condition, subjects entered a VR environment in which they were riding a boat on a river. Subjects were able to look around in a 360° VE while nature sounds were played through headphones. However, they were unable to interact with the VR world in any other way in this passive scenario. In the active VR condition, an interactive component was added to the passive scenario. Subjects were provided with 120 targets at various points along the river, which they were instructed to hit by aiming their heads in the direction of the target and pressing a button on the keyboard to 'shoot' a ball. Subjects were challenged to hit as many targets as possible. In the control condition, subjects wore the same HMD but only observed a dark screen, and no sound was emitted through the headphones. Subjects received noxious electrical stimuli at random intervals during all conditions. EPs were extracted time locked to stimuli. Pain scores were reported after each condition using NRS (0–10). Active VR significantly decreased pain scores and EP amplitudes. Passive VR had no analgesic effect. Interestingly, age was significantly correlated to pain scores, with older subjects demonstrating larger effects of VR. Gender, game experience and susceptibility for immersion through the means of post-exposure questionnaire, did not influence VR analgesia.

Enea *et al.* (2014) researched the effect of hypnotic analgesia (HA) and VR on the reduction of experimental pain in a group of 120 female students. The participants wore a head-mounted display with active software SnowWorld. Three experimentally induced pain treatment conditions were analysed: VRD, HA, and HA + VRD in relieving finger-pressure pain. All 3 treatments were more effective compared to the control group (no analgesia or distraction), irrespective of whether it involved HA, VRD, or both (hypnosis and VR). Participants rated pain using NRS (0–10) and verbal descriptor scale (1–6). VRD reduced pain regardless of hypnotisability. Magora *et al.* (2006) explored the use of VR immersion method of distraction to control experimental ischemic pain in 20 healthy volunteers (20–62 years). They used HMD and 3D interactive software game, in which the subject used the joystick to destroy enemy aliens. Pain control with and without the application of VR exposure was compared. They were told that the pain they would feel is the result of pressure maintained continuously on the forearm by an inflated regular blood pressure cuff and the lack of circulation in blood vessels below the tourniquet. Participants reported pain intensity and pain unpleasantness using VAS ratings (0–10). Tolerance time to ischemia was significantly longer for VR conditions than for those without. Affective distress ratings of unpleasantness and of time spent thinking about pain were significantly lower during VR as compared with the control condition. There was a significant difference between male and female on their tolerance time of ischemia in both experiments. Men spent significantly more time on VR than women. The study found that as the pain was created by tourniquet and the pain was a result of nerve compression than muscular pain, the affective distress from the arm cuff pressure pain and progressive numbness that happened later than the initial discomfort forced participants to reach the tolerance level of between 4 and 20 min.

Karaman *et al.* (2019) investigated the effect of the VR application on experimental pain severity in 172 healthy individuals. 'Roller coasters', an application that gives the impression that people are moving in a speeding train, was watched with a smartphone located in a VR Box headset. All individuals in the experimental and control groups were experimentally subjected to pain for two minutes by inflating a blood pressure cuff. During the procedure, the volunteers in the experimental group watched the 'roller coasters', while those in the control group received no intervention. Participants measured pain using VAS. They found that VR was effective in reducing the level of pain. Hoffman *et al.* (2006) examined the difference in the magnitude of VR analgesia between different display quality VR helmets in 77 volunteers (18–23 years). They compared high tech (using an active involvement software), low tech and control with no VR. The study showed that high-tech helmets reduced pain more than low tech. Gutierrez-Maldonado *et al.* (2010) examined the presence, involvement and efficacy of a VR intervention on pain in 45 healthy individuals with the help of an IPQ (Igroup Presence Questionnaire). They discovered that the amount of VR 'spatial presence' (relation between the VE and the subject's own body) reported, correlated significantly and positively with pain threshold and tolerance, and negatively with ratings of most pain intensity, time estimation and catastrophising (anticipating pain). Gutierrez-Maldonado *et al.*'s (2010) study has picked up on one of the gaps in the field and included two cognitive behaviours of catastrophising and self-efficacy. They also used VR in a unique approach. The VR environment consisted of a stereoscopic figure representing pain, in the centre of a black screen, allowing participants to control their pain by controlling the subject. Participants were able to change the unpleasant figure, and accompanying sound, to a pleasant and quiet environment.

4.2. *Obstetrics and gynaecology*

There were limited studies on the impact of VR on pain management within the obstetrics & gynaecology field. This can be due to the complexity of recruiting patient sample and patients' restriction of movement (Deo *et al.*, 2021). In one of the early experiments within this field, VR was applied and assessed among 30 primiparity women having episiotomy repair under local anaesthetic (LA) (Jahanishoorab *et al.*, 2015). The VR equipment consisted of a video player connected to a pair of video glasses including the connection cables and one 3D film (IMAX Dolpine and Whales 3D 1080p). Video glasses include two miniature LCD viewing screens (for the right and left eyes) with two external headphones. The unit included an external remote control device. Pain perception was reported using numeric rating scale. The results indicated that the clinical use of VR with LAs can reduce pain during episiotomy repair more than LA alone. Another interesting result from this study was a reduction in the perceived pain period (subject's estimation of the time required for the episiotomy repair). Patients stated that the perceived repair time was less than 46% of the actual time spent.

In a study by Frey *et al.* (2019), VR showed to have analgesic effect in labour in a study of 27 patients. VR delivered via an HMD with active software was compared to unmedicated labour followed by the opposite condition in a crossover study. Researchers used Samsung GearVR (Samsung, San Jose, CA) head-mounted display powered by a Galaxy S7 phone, a hand control and noise-reducing headphones powered by a parallel S5 phone, the Ocean Rift (www.ocean-rift.com) scuba diving simulation with sounds of manatee calls and breathing underwater. Additional relaxing music was supplied from night-time sleep by Brain.fm (www.brain.fm). User input consisted of head tracking and a hand control that simulated taking underwater photos. Significant decreases in sensory pain were observed during VR using numeric rating scale. On the other hand, Smith *et al.*'s (2020) study showed no significant differences in pain scores and procedure success rates, and anxiety levels were observed in patients during external cephalic version in a study of 50 adult patients. The participants used HMD, Samsung Gear VR in combination with a Samsung Galaxy S8 smartphone and 'Sky Lights' software (an active form of VR custom designed for the study by ALO VR). Pain and anxiety were measured using a 101-point NRS questionnaire.

Deo *et al.* (2021) looked into the use of VR for acute pain in 40 adult patients undergoing outpatient hysteroscopy. Immersive and interactive video content was delivered to patients via a head-mounted display

(Oculus Go). The guided relaxation experience included viewing an 8-min video called 'Forest of Serenity' commissioned by St Giles Hospice, developed by Holosphere and narrated by Sir David Attenborough. Compared with standard care, women with VR intervention experienced less average pain and anxiety using the numeric rating scale.

4.3. *Burns*

VRD was used to reduce burns patients' discomfort and pain from early days of VR introduction. One of the first studies was done by Hoffman *et al.* (2000), which has looked into using 3D VR as an adjunctive pain control and highlighted the need for non-pharmaceutical analgesic interventions. VR relaxation has been shown to increase pain intensity for participants receiving VR with morphine during burn wound dressing changes. VR relaxation sequence prepared by psychologists based on hypnotherapy was used. While VRD is effective for reducing pain during burn wound care, VR relaxation may not deliver the same result. The level of immersion was not examined in this study (Konstantatos *et al.*, 2009).

VRD aids analgesia during joint flexibility exercises of burn victims in 39 adult patients (Soltani *et al.*, 2018). Participants were equipped with VR goggles with active software (the participants moved a computer mouse to control perspective and aim snowballs in the icy canyon VE), while performing unassisted active range of movement (ROM) exercises both with and without VRD in a randomised order. A 0–100 GRS was used to assess the pain. A GRS rating of the amount of 'fun' during stretching served as a measure of positive experience. VR reduced pain perception for worst pain, pain unpleasantness and time spent thinking about pain. However, patients did not show greater ROM during VR. These results were replicated by Carrougher *et al.* (2009).

The technology is used during burns patients' dressing change. Guo *et al.* (2015) used VR in modifying pain perception during dressing changes in patients with hand injury. 98 adult participants were given ultra-high-resolution 3D glasses projecting a 3D film. Significant difference in VAS scores was observed after the dressing change. Importantly, the correlation between the sense of involvement in a VE and pain level during the dressing was statistically significant. VRD can effectively alleviate pain among patients with a hand injury undergoing a dressing change. Better results can be obtained by increasing the sense of involvement in a VE. McSherry *et al.* (2018) looked into the application of immersive VR (IVR) to decrease opioid use during painful wound care procedures. A study of 18 adult patients compared IVR and opioids vs opioids alone in adult patients undergoing dressing changes. IVR consisted of VR goggles, headphones and an active software. IVR reduced the amount of opioid medication administered during painful wound care procedures by 39% when IVR was used compared with no IVR.

4.4. *General surgery*

Ding *et al.* (2019) examined VR as a distraction tool in decreasing pain during daily dressing changes following haemorrhoid surgery in 182 adult patients. HMD with an immersive active VR software was used to achieve the virtual distraction activity (SnowWorld). The control group received the standard pharmacological analgesic intervention during dressing change and a VRG received VRD during dressing change plus standard pharmacological analgesic intervention. There was no significant difference in mean pain scores (visual analogue score) prior to and after the dressing change procedure between the two groups. However, the mean pain scores during the first dressing change were significantly lower in the VRG compared with the control group. Haisley *et al.* (2020) looked into the application of VR headset with mindfulness/meditation software to alleviate postoperative pain in 52 adult patients after benign UGI surgery (mean age 64.5 years). Researchers used wireless VR headset with mindfulness/meditation application. Patients in VRG reported low pain, anxiety and nausea scores while using the device. However, no difference in pain perception between the two groups was observed.

4.5. *Orthopaedics*

Gianola *et al.* (2020) conducted an RCT examining the effects of early VR-based rehabilitation in 85 adult patients with total knee arthroplasty. VR rehabilitation was compared with traditional rehabilitation. A statistically significant improvement was present in the global proprioception.

However, there was no statistically significant difference in pain reduction (using visual analogue score), the health-related quality of life, the global perceived effect, the functional independent measure, the drugs assumption, the isometric strength of quadriceps and hamstrings, and the flexion range of motion.

Huang *et al.* (2020) explored the effects of immersive virtual reality (IVR) therapy on intravenous patient-controlled sedation (PCS) during orthopaedic surgery under regional anaesthesia in a sample of 50 adults. They used either a Samsung Gear VR HMD (Samsung, Korea) or the Oculus Rift Development Kit 2 (Oculus Inc, California, USA) HMDs. Both HMDs feature a large field of view and high-quality display; both blocked the user's view of their immediate environment. The software allowed subjects to float along a procedurally generated three-dimensional river. Authors used quality of recovery score (QoR 40). IVR plus propofol PCS and propofol PCS alone were compared. IVR was well tolerated but did not decrease the overall sedation requirement.

4.6. *Urology*

Walker *et al.* (2014) examined the efficacy of VRD in the reduction of pain and anxiety during cystoscopy on 43 adult patients. Authors used VR helmet and trackball hand controller with SnowWorld software where participants were tasked to shoot snowballs at penguins, robots and igloos. Participants used VAS. Intraprocedural anxiety, average pain, worst pain and time spent thinking about pain were higher in the VR group (VRG), however, without statistical significance. There were no adverse events reported including nausea or dizziness.

Basak *et al.* (2020) explored VR's role as a distraction-based relief of pain associated with peripheral intravenous catheterisation in 120 adult patients. VR goggles were projecting a 3D video. After mobile phone placement in the pull chamber at the front side of the VR goggle, it was attached by a headband. Participants used a visual analogue score. The authors found that the use of cards containing distracting optical illusion pictures and playing 3D videos with VR goggles during PIC insertion in adult patients were effective methods of pain reduction. Furthermore, the study yielded a high level of patient satisfaction.

4.7. *Cardiothoracic*

Bruno *et al.* (2020) examined the use of VR-assisted conscious sedation during transcatheter aortic valve implantation (TAVI) on 32 elderly patients. Patients could choose one of the following videos: nature scenery, an aquarium, flying over a green landscape, diving underwater or walking through a calm forest. The VR intervention group reported significantly less anxiety after the procedure than patients randomised to control using visual analogue score. In the intervention group, 93.8% would use VR during TAVI again. Nausea and vomiting did not occur more frequently compared to control. Cacau *et al.* (2013) explored the use of VR as an intervention tool post cardiac surgery on 60 adult patients. Patients allocated to VRG were treated twice a day (in the morning and afternoon), performing the same techniques than conventional treatment, however the motor exercise was performed using VR. The length of stay was reduced by 3 days in patients of VRG, also a 6-min walking distance was increased by 50 m in the VRG.

4.8. *Dental*

Tanja-Dijkstra *et al.* (2014) explored the role of VR in dental practice on 69 adult patients. They used an HMD projecting a 3D VE, depicted a coastal path, complete with sea, beach and field areas. They examined active VR vs passive VR vs control. Wireless VR headset with a mindfulness/meditation application pre-installed was given to participants. The active VRG experienced a higher level of presence (immersion) than the passive VRG. Participants used a dental anxiety score. VRD intervention did not only impact the experience of a simulated aversive event, it also reduced the vividness of memories of such an event a week later. This study thus suggests that VRDs can be considered as a relevant intervention for cycles of care in which people's previous experiences affect their behaviour for future events. If a dental patient, e.g. has a more positive experience of a treatment due to the VRD intervention, that patient might have less vivid memories and as a consequence might be less likely to postpone a future dental visit. Furman *et al.* (2009) looked at VRD for pain control during periodontal scaling and root planning procedures in a sample of 38. VR was compared with watching a movie and a control group. Pain scores measured with visual analogue score were significantly lower in the VRG compared with the movie group and controls.

4.9. *Mixed*

Spiegel *et al.* (2019) conducted an RCT with 120 adult patients on medical, orthopaedic, gastrointestinal or psychiatric wards in the USA. Patients in the experimental group received a library of 21 VR experiences administered using a Samsung Gear Oculus headset; control patients viewed specialised television programming to promote health and wellness. VR yielded a reduction in pain vs control using numeric rating scale.

4.10. *Conclusion*

There is a good body of evidence to support the use of VR in pain management in clinical practice. It acts as a good distraction tool. Overall, no adverse outcomes were reported. No difference in nausea and dizziness between VR and control groups was observed. Active software has been shown to be superior to the passive one. Complete immersion with visual and audio stimulation replaced by VR environment is important. The results were similar in different age groups. The use of VR in postoperative pain is limited. The main areas of application would be in short procedures where it not only delivers better pain management but also decreases the need for pharmaceutical analgesia and increases patient satisfaction.

4.11. *Limitation*

One of the main limitations of the reviewed studies was the small number of participants in the majority of the studies, and the fact that all of the participants were from a particular population such as young female students (Weeth *et al.*, 2017). All of them were performed in a single centre, sometimes by a single professional administering treatment (e.g. Deo *et al.*, 2021; Ding *et al.*, 2019). From the design point of view, it seems impossible to perform a blind study as it is obvious to participants and assessors to what group a participant belongs (e.g. Huang *et al.*, 2020). Also, it is not possible to be ambitious in research design, when the sample is from a pool of patients as the studies need to be patient-centred, adhering to patients' treatment and safety first. When using healthy patients, the flexibility in research design increases, but there are arguments against the findings not being generalisable to the patient pool due to the sample being healthy individuals (e.g. Lier *et al.*, 2020). There were limitations from software and hardware used in studies, as some were selected due to availability or convenience. For example, SnowWorld, a software developed by University of Washington HITLab, was one of the most popular programmes used in VR studies (Waker *et al.*, 2014; Hoffman *et al.*, 2006, 2008). Some studies reported patients to be uncomfortable with VR technology (e.g. Gianola *et al.*, 2020), and some reported that realism was not achieved (Weeth *et al.*, 2017).

For pain evaluation, most of the studies used visual/numeric analogue scores or alternatives, which were self-reported by participants. This results in a subjective bias (e.g. Karaman *et al.*, 2019). Many factors that are highlighted in literature as having a correlation or moderating effect on pain perception were not considered in many studies, such as existing pain experience, patients' pain threshold or perceived self-efficacy (e.g. Karaman *et al.*, 2019; Weeth *et al.*, 2017). This limitation is addressed in some of the later studies, such as Lier *et al.* (2020), who excluded participants suffering from acute or chronic pain at the time of the experiment.

5. What the Future Holds?

Based on the existing exploration of academic literature, for an effective delivery of VR in acute pain management, two factors are addressed: first, the main user group benefiting from intervention needs to be identified; second, the most appropriate VR technology needs to be selected.

5.1. *VR user group*

To address the question of who benefits from VR the most, what is highlighted in the present work is that VR is proven effective for certain patient groups, such as burn patients. However, in other fields such as obstetrics and gynaecology or experimental, there were contradictory results. For instance, Smith *et al.* (2020) indicated no significant difference for the perceived pain between patients using VR and the control group. Enea *et al.*'s (2014) findings indicated no significant difference in perceived pain between HA, VRD or both. In orthopaedics, Huang *et al.* (2020) indicated that although VR resulted in more pain tolerance, it didn't decrease the sedation requirement. These contradictory outcomes can be due to the sample characteristics. This is highlighted in some of the studies, for instance, Magora *et al.* (2006), found that men showed more tolerance than women while interacting with a 3D interactive software game, in which the subject used the joystick to destroy enemy alien. Gutierrez-Maldonado *et al.*'s (2010) findings indicated participants' pain thresholds play an important role on their level of immersion and pain perception.

In order to identify the most suitable target patient for VR intervention, academic work needs to explore factors such as age, gaming experience, behavioural factors such as attitude, self-efficacy and prior and existing pain experience and threshold. Lessons can be learned from computer–human interaction literature and technological behaviour. It is also essential to evaluate presence to get a better insight into patients' behaviour towards VR intervention. This is not surprising if the difference in patients' response to the VR intervention is due to them not perceiving a similar level of presence in the VR environment. Furthermore, research needs to look into user engagement and involvement and how this can impact VR's effectiveness. If users are not involved but immersed, would they still have a positive experience using VR in pain management as observed in Gutierrez-Maldonado *et al.* (2010) or would involvement be part of active participation and inseparable from presence?

5.2. *VR application and technology*

For the user group that interacts and immerses into the VR environment, the effectiveness of the intervention increases. But, would VR be deemed effective when reducing patients' pain or discomfort or can the technology have a longer-term impact on patients' pain perception, catastrophising, attitude, etc.? Majority of the studies used VR platforms to create an active or passive distraction environment for sufferers. Some studies looked into the inclusion of other interventions such as HA or sedation. Only one study by Gutierrez-Maldonado *et al.* (2010) used VR to psychologically manipulate users' perception and feeling towards and experience of pain. VR needs to be used more creatively, to not only provide a short-term solution to patients' pain but a long-term intervention for patients' change in attitude towards pain and factors impacting pain perception.

New headsets are becoming lighter in weight, which results in more comfort for the user. Users can wear headsets for longer periods of time. This longer usability is also facilitated by changes in the lenses used in VR headsets, older models include single focal lengths, which means users need to go cross-eyed to focus on items that are outside of that length. Oculus is introducing a new type of lens that adjusts the focus point dynamically. Advanced headsets (such as Varjo and Pimax) also contain a better resolution, up to four times better than the older models. There has been a big shift in the user interface of VR headsets and more convergence. New models include better design, some new headsets use cameras on the headset to track users' hands and movement and eliminate the need for controllers. Forbes reports that most popular VR applications nowadays take control of users' senses of sight and hearing in order to provide users with total immersion. The advancement in VR interface not only results in more 'realism', which can increase user immersion, but also increase the usability of this technology. For example, headsets that allow patients' hand movement to be detected can be used in rehabilitation and result in a better sense of presence in the VE. Companies develop new hardware and software to enhance the sense of presence and create a more real experience. Headsets are being replaced with VR glasses, an advanced example is Hololens by Microsoft, which is a mixed-reality holographic device that gives users abilities to be engaged in the virtual world as well as the physical world. However, in order to bring this technology to the healthcare industry, and make this widely available to patients, the cost, accessibility, compatibility, ease of use and comfort need to be taken into consideration. This is essential for turning it into a reality in patient care, rather than it remaining a mere dream.

References

Ahmadpour, N., Randall, H., Choksi, H., Gao, A., Vaughan, C. & Poronnik, P. (2019) Virtual reality interventions for acute and chronic pain management. *The International Journal of Biochemistry & Cell Biology*, 114, 105568.

Ahn, S. J. (2011) Embodied experiences in immersive virtual environments: Effects on pro-environmental attitude and behavior. Doctoral Dissertation, Stanford University, Palo Alto, CA.

Ahn, D. & Shin, D. H. (2016) Observers versus agents: Divergent associations of video versus game use with empathy and social connectedness. *Information Technology and People*, 29(3), 1.

Asghari Moghaddam, M. A. (2014) Changing the concept of pain over time. *Biannual Journal of Clinical Psychology and Personality*, 13(2), 165–172.

Basak, C., Qin, S. & Oconnell, M. (2020) Differential effects of cognitive training modules in healthy aging and mild cognitive impairment: A comprehensive meta-analysis of randomized controlled trials. *Psychology and Aging*, 35(2), 220.

Bhatt, G. (2004) Bringing virtual reality for commercial Web sites. *International Journal of Human-Computer Studies*, 60(1), 1–15.

Blount, R. L., Powers, S. W., Cotter, M. W., Swan, S. & Free, K. (1994) Making the system work. Training paediatric oncology patients to cope and their parents to coach them during BMA/LP procedures. *Behavior Modification*, 18, 6–31.

Brekke, M., Hjortdahl, P. & Kvien, T. (2003) Changes in self-efficacy and health status over 5 years: A longitudinal observational study of 306 patients with rheumatoid arthritis. *Arthritis & Rheumatism*, 49, 342–348.

Bruno, R. R., *et al.* (2020) Virtual reality-assisted conscious sedation during transcatheter aortic valve implantation: A randomised pilot study. *EuroIntervention*, 16(12), e1014–e1020.

Cacau, L. A. P., Oliveira, G. U., Maynard, L. G., Araújo Filho, A. A., Silva, W. M., Jr, Cerqueria Neto, M. L., Antoniolli, A. R. & Santana-Filho, V. J. (2013) The use of the virtual reality as intervention tool in the postoperative of cardiac surgery. *Revista Brasileira de Cirurgia Cardiovascular*, 28(2), 281–289. doi: 10.5935/1678–9741.20130039.

Carrougher, G. J., Hoffman, H. G., Nakamura, D., Lezotte, D., Soltani, M., Leahy, L., Engrav, L. H. & Patterson, D. R. (2009) The effect of virtual reality on pain and range of motion in adults with burn injuries. *Journal of Burn Care & Research*, 30(5), 785–791.

Cohen, L., Blount, R., Cohen, R., Schaen, E. & Zaff, J. (1999) Comparative study of distraction versus topical anesthesia for pediatric pain management during immunizations. *Health Psychology*, 18, 591–598.

Dascal, J., Reid, M., IsHak, W. W., Spiegel, B., Recacho, J., Rosen, B. & Danovitch, I. (2017) Virtual reality and medical inpatients: A systematic review of randomized, controlled trials. *Innovations in Clinical Neuroscience*, 14(1–2), 14–21.

Deo, N., Khan, K. S., Mak, J., Allotey, J., Gonzalez Carreras, F. J., Fusari, G. & Benn, J. (2021) Virtual reality for acute pain in outpatient hysteroscopy: A randomised controlled trial. *British Journal of Obstetrics and Gynaecology*, 128(1), 87–95.

Ding, L., Hua, H., Zhu, H., Zhu, S., Lu, J., Zhao, K. & Xu, Q. (2020) Effects of virtual reality on relieving postoperative pain in surgical patients: A systematic review and meta-analysis. *International Journal of Surgery*, 82, 87–94.

Donegan, M. L., Stefanini, F., Meira, T., Gordon, J. A., Fusi, S. & Siegelbaum, S. A. (2020) Coding of social novelty in the hippocampal CA2 region and its disruption and rescue in a 22q11.2 microdeletion mouse model. *Nature Neuroscience*, 23(11), 1365–1375.

Enea, V., Dafinoiu, I., Opriş, D. & David, D. (2014) Effects of hypnotic analgesia and virtual reality on the reduction of experimental pain among high and low hypnotizables. *International Journal of Clinical and Experimental Hypnosis*, 62(3), 360–377.

Faruki, A., Nguyen, T., Proeschel, S., Levy, N., Yu, J., Ip, V., Mueller, A., Banner-Goodspeed, V. & O'Gara, B. (2019) Virtual reality as an adjunct to anesthesia in the operating room. *Trials*, 20(1), 782.

Felemban, O. M., Alshamrani, R. M., Aljeddawi, D. H., *et al.* (2021) Effect of virtual reality distraction on pain and anxiety during infiltration anesthesia in pediatric patients: A randomized clinical trial. *BMC Oral Health*, 21, 321.

Ferrer-Garcia, M., Gutiérrez-Maldonado, J. & Riva, G. (2013) Virtual reality based treatments in eating disorders and obesity: A review. *Journal of Contemporary Psychotherapy*, 43(4), 207–221.

Fowler-Kerry, S. & Lander, J. (1987) Management of injection pain in children. *Pain*, 30, 69–75.

Frey, D. P., Bauer, M. E., Bell, C. L., Low, L. K., Hassett, A. L., Cassidy, R. B., Boyer, K. D. & Sharar, S. R. (2019) Virtual reality analgesia in labor: The VRAIL pilot study-A preliminary randomized controlled trial suggesting benefit of immersive virtual reality analgesia in unmedicated laboring women. *Anesthesia and Analgesia*, 128(6), e93–e96.

Furman, E., Jasinevicius, T. R., Bissada, N. F., Victoroff, K. Z., Skillicorn, R. & Buchner, M. (2009) Virtual reality distraction for pain control during periodontal scaling and root planning procedures. *Journal of the American Dental Association*, 140(12), 1508–1516.

Gianola, S., Stucovitz, E., Castellini, G., Mascali, M., Vanni, F., Tramacere, I., Banfi, G. & Tornese, D. (2020) Effects of early virtual reality-based rehabilitation in patients with total knee arthroplasty: A randomized controlled trial. *Medicine (Baltimore)*, 99(7), e19136.

Gloth, F. M., 3rd, Scheve, A. A., Stober, C. V., Chow, S. & Prosser, J. (2001) The functional pain scale: Reliability, validity, and responsiveness in an elderly population. *Journal of the American Medical Directors Association*, 2(3), 110–114.

Gutierrez-Maldonado, J., Gutierrez-Martinez, O., Loreto, D., Peñaloza, C. & Nieto, R. (2010) Presence, involvement and efficacy of a virtual reality intervention on pain. *Studies in Health Technology and Informatics*, 154(1), 97–101.

Guo, C., Deng, H. & Yang, Y. (2015) Effect of virtual reality distraction on pain among patients with hand injury undergoing dressing change. *Journal of Clinical Nursing*, 24(1–2), 115–120.

Haisley, K. R., Straw, O. J., Müller, D. T., Antiporda, M. A., Zihni, A. M., Reavis, K. M., Bradley, D. D. & Dunst, C. M. (2020) Feasibility of implementing a virtual reality program as an adjuvant tool for peri-operative pain control; results of a randomized controlled trial in minimally invasive foregut surgery. *Complementary Therapies in Medicine*, 49, 102356.

Handa, M., Aul, E. G. & Bajaj, S. (2012) Immersive technology — uses, challenges and opportunities. *International Journal of Computing and Business Research*, 1–11.

Hodges, L., Rothbaum, B. O., Kooper, R., Opdyke, D., Meyer, T., de Graaf, J. J. & Williford, J. S. (1994) Presence as the defining factor in a VR application. Georgia Institute of Technology.

Hoffman, H. G. (2004) Virtual reality therapy. *Scientific American*, 291(2), 58–65.

Hoffman, H. G., Patterson, D. R. & Carrougher, G. J. (2000) Use of virtual reality for adjunctive treatment of adult burn pain during physical therapy: A controlled study. *The Clinical Journal of Pain*, 16(3), 244–250.

Hoffman, H. G., Richards, T. L., Van Oostrom, T., Coda, B. A., Jensen, M. P., Blough, D. K. & Sharar, S. R. (2007) The analgesic effects of opioids and immersive virtual reality distraction: Evidence from subjective and functional brain imaging assessments. *Anesthesia and Analgesia*, 105(6), 1776–1783.

Hone-Blanchet, A., Wensing, T. & Fecteau, S. (2014) The use of virtual reality in craving assessment and cue-exposure therapy in substance use disorders. *Frontiers in Human Neuroscience*, 8, 844.

Huang, K. H., Rupprecht, P., Frank, T., *et al.* (2020) A virtual reality system to analyze neural activity and behavior in adult zebrafish. *Nature Methods*, 17, 343–351.

Inan, G. & Inal, S. (2019) The impact of 3 different distraction techniques on the pain and anxiety levels of children during venipuncture: A clinical trial. *Clinical Journal of Pain*, 35(2), 140–147.

JahaniShoorab, N., Ebrahimzadeh Zagami, S., Nahvi, A., Mazluom, S. R., Golmakani, N., Talebi, M. & Pabarja, F. (2015) The effect of virtual reality on pain in primiparity women during episiotomy repair: A randomized clinical trial. *Iranian Journal of Medical Sciences*, 40(3), 219–224.

Jensen, M. P., Turner, J. A., Romano, J. M. & Karoly, P. (1991) Coping with chronic pain: A critical review of literature. *Pain*, 47, 249–283.

Jerdan, S. W., Grindle, M. & van Woerden, H. C. (2018) Head-mounted virtual reality and mental health: Critical review of current research. *JMIR Serious Games*, 6, e14.

Jin, C., Feng, Y., Ni, Y. & Shan, Z. (2018) Virtual reality intervention in postoperative rehabilitation after total knee arthroplasty: A prospective and randomized controlled clinical trial.

Johnson, M. H. (2005) How does distraction work in the management of pain? *Current Pain and Headache Reports*, 9(2), 90–95.

Karaman, D., Erol, F., Yılmaz, D. & Dikmen, Y. (2019) Investigation of the effect of the virtual reality application on experimental pain severity in healthy. *Revista da Associação Médica Brasileira*, 65, 446–451.

Keefe, F. J., Rumble, M. E., Scipio, C. D., Giordano, L. A. & Perri, L. M. (2004) Psychological aspects of persistent pain: Current state of the science. *The Journal of Pain*, 5, 195–211.

Klein, L. R. (2003) Creating virtual product experiences: The role of telepresence. *Journal of Interactive Marketing*, 17(1), 41–55. doi: 10.1002/dir. 10046.

Konstantatos, A. H., Angliss, M., Costello, V., Cleland, H. & Stafrace, S. (2009) Predicting the effectiveness of virtual reality relaxation on pain and anxiety when added to PCA morphine in patients having burns dressings changes. *Burns*, 35(4), 491–499.

Li, B. J., Bailenson, J. N., Pines, A., Greenleaf, W. J. & Williams, L. M. (2017) A public database of immersive VR videos with corresponding ratings of arousal, valence, and correlations between head movements and self report measures. *Frontiers in Psychology*, 8.

Li, A., Montaño, Z., Chen, V. J. & Gold, J. I. (2011) Virtual reality and pain management: Current trends and future directions. *Pain Management*, 1, 147–157.

Li, L., Yu, F., Shi, D., Shi, J., Tian, Z., Yang, J., *et al.* (2017) Application of virtual reality technology in clinical medicine. *American Journal of Translational Research*, 9(9), 3867–3880.

Lier, E. J., Oosterman, J. M., Assmann, R., *et al.* (2020) The effect of virtual reality on evoked potentials following painful electrical stimuli and subjective pain. *Scientific Reports*, 10, 9067.

Loreto-Quijada, D., Gutiérrez-Maldonado, J., Nieto, R., Gutiérrez-Martínez, O., Ferrer-García, M., Saldaña, C., Fusté-Escolano, A. & Liutsko, L. (2014) Differential effects of two virtual reality interventions: Distraction versus pain control. *Cyberpsychology, Behavior, and Social Networking*, 17(6), 353–358.

Magora, F., Cohen, S., Shochina, M. & Dayan, E. (2006) Virtual reality immersion method of distraction to control experimental ischemic pain. *Israel Medical Association Journal*, 8, 261–265.

Walker, M. R., Kallingal, G. J. S., Musser, J. E., Folen, R., Stetz, M. C. & Clark, J. Y. (2014) Treatment efficacy of virtual reality distraction in the reduction of pain and anxiety during cystoscopy. *Military Medicine*, 179(8), 891–896.

Maples-Keller, J. L., Bunnell, B. E., Kim, S. J. & Rothbaum, B. O. (2017) The use of virtual reality technology in the treatment. *Harvard Review of Psychiatry*, 25(3), 103–113.

Marks, R. B., Sibley, S. D. & Ben Arbaugh, J. (2005) A structural equation model of predictors for effective online learning. *Journal of Management Education*, 29(4), 531–563.

Massetti, T., da Silva, T. D., Crocetta, T. B., Guarnieri, R., de Freitas, B. L., Bianchi Lopes, P., *et al.* (2018) The clinical utility of virtual reality in neurorehabilitation: A systematic review. *Journal of Central Nervous System Disease*.

Matheve, T., Bogaerts, K. & Timmermans, A. (2020) Virtual reality distraction induces hypoalgesia in patients with chronic low back pain: A randomized controlled trial. *Journal of NeuroEngineering and Rehabilitation*, 17, 55.

McSherry, T., Atterbury, M., Gartner, S., Helmold, E., Searles, D. M. & Schulman, C. (2018) Randomized, crossover study of immersive virtual reality to decrease opioid use during painful wound care procedures in adults. *Journal of Burn Care and Research*, 39(2), 278–285.

Meldrum, M. (2003) A capsule history of pain management. *The Journal of the American Medical Association*, 290(18), 2470–2475.

Melzack, R. & Wall, P. D. (1996) Pain mechanisms: A new theory: A gate control system modulates sensory input from the skin before it evokes pain perception and response. *Pain Forum*, 5(1), 3–11.

Mitrousia, V. & Giotakos, O. (2016) Virtual reality therapy in anxiety disorders. *Psychiatriki*, 27(4), 276–286.

North, M. M., North, S. M. & Coble, J. R. (1997) Virtual reality therapy: An effective treatment for psychological disorders. Virtual reality in neuro-psycho-physiology: Cognitive, clinical and methodological issues in assessment and rehabilitation. p. 13.

Plotzky, C., Lindwedel, U., Sorber, M., Loessl, B., König, P., Kunze, C., Kugler, C. & Meng, M. (2021) Virtual reality simulations in nurse education: A systematic mapping review. *Nurse Education Today*, 101, 104868.

Quartana, P. J., Campbell, C. M. & Edwards, R. R. (2009) Pain catastrophizing: A critical review. *Expert Review of Neurotherapeutics*, 9(5), 745–758.

Ragusa, J. M. & Bochenek, G. M. (2001) Collaborative virtual design environments. *Communications of the ACM*, 44(12), 40–43.

Schütze, R., Rees, C., Preece, M. & Schutze, M. (2010) Low mindfulness predicts pain catastrophizing in a fear-avoidance model of chronic pain. *Pain*, 148(1), 120–127.

Scott, J. & Huskisson, E. C. (1976) Graphic representation of pain. *Pain*, 2(2), 175–184.

Seyed Esfahani, M., Heydari Khajehpour, S., Roushan-Easton, G. & Howell, R. D. (2022) A framework for successful adoption of surgical innovation. *Surgical Innovation*.

Sharifpour, S., Manshaee, G. & Sajjadian, I. (2020) Effects of virtual reality therapy on perceived pain intensity, anxiety, catastrophising and self-efficacy among adolescents with cancer. *Counselling and Psychotherapy Research*, 21(3), 218–226.

Sharar, S. R., Carrougher, G. J., Nakamura, D., Hoffman, H. G., Blough, D. K. & Patterson, D. R. (2007) Factors influencing the efficacy of virtual reality distraction analgesia during postburn physical therapy: Preliminary results from 3 ongoing studies. *Archives of Physical Medicine and Rehabilitation*, 88(12 Suppl 2), S43–S49.

Sharar, S. R., Carrougher, G. J., Selzer, K., O'Donnell, F., Vavilala, M. S. & Lee, L. A. (2002) A comparison of oral transmucosal fentanyl citrate and oral oxycodone for pediatric outpatient wound care. *Journal of Burn Care and Rehabilitation*, 23(1), 27–31.

Shin, D., Biocca, F. & Choo, H. (2013) Erratum: Exploring the user experience of 3D virtual learning environments. *Behaviour & Information Technology*, 32(2), 203–214.

Slifer, K. J., Tucker, C. L. & Dahlquist, L. M. (2002) Helping children and caregivers cope with repeated invasive procedures: How are we doing? *Journal of Clinical Psychology in Medical Settings*, 9, 131–152.

Smith, V., Warty, R. R., Sursas, J. A., Payne, O., Nair, A., Krishnan, S., da Silva Costa, F., Wallace, E. M. & Vollenhoven, B. (2020) The effectiveness of virtual reality in managing acute pain and anxiety for medical inpatients: Systematic review. *Journal of Medical Internet Research*, 22(11), e17980.

Soltani, M., Drever, S. A., Hoffman, H. G., Sharar, S. R., Wiechman, S. A., Jensen, M. P. & Patterson, D. R. (2018) Virtual reality analgesia for burn joint flexibility: A randomized controlled trial. *Rehabilitation Psychology*, 63(4), 487–494.

Spiegel, B., Fuller, G., Lopez, M., Dupuy, T., Noah, B., Howard, A., Albert, M., Tashjian, V., Lam, R., Ahn, J., Dailey, F., Rosen, B. T., Vrahas, M., Little, M., Garlich, J., Dzubur, E., IsHak, W. & Danovitch, I. (2019) Virtual reality for management of pain in hospitalized patients: A randomized comparative effectiveness trial. *PLoS One*, 14(8), e0219115.

Sra, M., Xu, X. & Maes P. (2018) BreathVR: Leveraging breathing as a directly controlled interface for virtual reality games. In: *Proceedings of the 2018 CHI Conference on Human Factors in Computing Systems*. Association for Computing Machinery, New York, NY, USA, Paper 340, pp. 1–12.

Steuer, J. (1992) Defining virtual reality: Dimensions determining telepresence. *Journal of Communication*, 42(4), 73–93.

Sullivan, M., Thorn, B., Haythornthwaite, J., Keefe, F., Martin, M., Bradley, L. & Lefebvre, J. (2001) Theoretical perspectives on the relation between catastrophizing and pain. *Clinical Journal of Pain*, 17, 52–64.

Taenzer, P., Melzack, R. & Jeans, M. E. (1986) Influence of psychological factors on postoperative pain, mood and analgesic requirements. *Pain*, 24, 331–342.

Tanja-Dijkstra, K., Pahl, S., White, M. P., Andrade, J., Qian, C., Bruce, M., May, J. & Moles, D. R. (2014) Improving dental experiences by using virtual reality distraction: A simulation study. *PLoS One*, 9(3), e91276.

Toyoda, R., Russo Abegão, F., Gill, S., *et al.* (2021) Drivers of immersive virtual reality adoption intention: A multi-group analysis in chemical industry settings. *Virtual Reality*, 1–12.

Turner, J. A., Holtzman, S. & Mancl, L. (2007) Mediators, moderators and predictors of therapeutic change in cognitive-behavioral therapy for chronic pain. *Pain*, 127, 276–286.

Walker, M. R., Kallingal, G. J., Musser, J. E., Folen, R., Stetz, M. C. & Clark, J. Y. (2014) Treatment efficacy of virtual reality distraction in the reduction of pain and anxiety during cystoscopy. *Military Medicine*, 179(8), 891–896.

Wade, J. B., Price, D., Hamer, R. M., Schwartz, S. M. & Hart, R. P. (1990) An emotional component analysis of chronic pain. *Pain*, 40, 303–310.

Weeth, A., Mühlberger, A. & Shiban, Y. (2017) Was it less painful for knights? Influence of appearance on pain perception. *European Journal of Pain*, 21(10), 1756–1762.

Wismeijer, A. A. & Vingerhoets, A. J. (2005) The use of virtual reality and audiovisual eyeglass systems as adjunct analgesic techniques: A review of the literature. *Annals of Behavioral Medicine*, 30(3), 268–278.

Witmer, B. G. & Singer, M. J. (1998) Measuring presence in virtual environments: A presence questionnaire. *Presence: Teleoperators and Virtual Environments*, 7(3), 225–240.

Yang, H., Chu, H., Kao, C., Chiu, H., Tseng, I., Tseng, P., *et al.* (2019) Development and effectiveness of virtual interactive working memory training for older people with mild cognitive impairment: A single-blind randomised controlled trial. *Age and Ageing*, 48, 519–525.

Zeltzer, L. K., Dolgin, M., LeBaron, S. & LeBaron, C. (1991) A randomized, controlled study of behavioral intervention for chemotherapy distress in children with cancer. *Pediatrics*, 88, 34–42.

https://doi.org/10.1142/9781800614192_0008

Chapter 8

ALAMEDA: Towards the Technology-Enabled Optimisation of Brain Healthcare Continuum

Valentina Tageo* and the ALAMEDA H2020 Project Consortium

Wise Angle Consulting SL, Spain

vtageo@wiseangle.es

ALAMEDA is an international and multidisciplinary research project funded by the EU in the frame of the H2020 Research and Innovation Framework Programme aiming to bridge the early diagnosis and treatment gap of brain diseases via smart, connected, proactive and evidence-based technological interventions. The present chapter illustrates the overall integrated, multidisciplinary and participatory approach to brain healthcare that ALAMEDA promotes by developing and testing the next generation AI-based healthcare support systems. Innovative technologies and models are meant to provide personalised disease monitoring as well as rehabilitation and treatment assessment for patients with Parkinson's disease, multiple sclerosis and stroke (PMSS). This will support the design of outcome-driven interventions, allow that situations likely to aggravate can be predicted and boost the transition to value-based healthcare models.

As the project is still ongoing, the chapter specifically focuses on a thorough overview of the respective care journeys, focusing specific attention on current healthcare service organisation and provision, their degree of multidisciplinarity and integration as well as digitalisation and personalisation. In addition, the authors dive into the three national contexts where the ALAMEDA solutions are being tested and discuss current workloads and procedures, the interconnectedness of services and providers at the local level and the efforts currently being made to give increasing weight to patients' preferences in medical decision-making. From the insights obtained via desk search and direct consultation with the involved clinicians, the document points out the enabling and potentially hindering factors for the future development and deployment of the solutions locally. Last, the chapter describes the end users' adopted engagement strategy and how the concepts and models from other research projects (such as MULTI-ACT) and well-established practices in medical settings (i.e. shared decision-making) are interpreted and adapted into the context of the innovative value-based healthcare digital transformation framework promoted by the ALAMEDA consortium.

1. Introduction

ALAMEDA is an international collaborative and multidisciplinary research project funded by the European Union in the frame of the Horizon 2020 Research and Innovation Framework Programme aiming to bridge the early diagnosis and treatment gap of brain diseases via smart, connected, proactive and evidence-based technological interventions. A strong consortium of 15 partners, comprising medical specialists, health informatics and AI researchers, medical software developers, vendors and healthcare market experts, with a budget of ~6 MEUR started working on January 2021, in an effort to research, develop and exploit the next generation of personalised AI healthcare support systems that improve remote patient monitoring and treatment assessment of Parkinson's disease (PD), multiple sclerosis (MS) and stroke patients. ALAMEDA acknowledges that the care of patients with brain disorders is complex, and manifestations of certain diseases could worsen over time and seriously impair the quality of life of patients and their caregivers.

Through the use of artificial intelligence (AI) healthcare support systems, the project aims to provide personalised disease monitoring as well as rehabilitation and treatment assessment for patients with PD, MS and stroke, to ensure that interventions are effective and that situations likely to aggravate can be predicted. The design and validation of such solutions entail the identification of meaningful use cases and health outcomes that can provide solid evidence for the application of the principles of value-based healthcare. Furthermore, patient engagement across the Research & Innovation (R&I) process and high attention to usability and user-friendliness aspects play a pivotal role in maximising the acceptance of technologies that are likely to transform care pathways. For this reason, the ALAMEDA AI-based personalised prediction, prevention, and intervention approach is being deployed and tested in three real-world pilots in Greece, Italy and Romania with the activation of local community groups of patients, caregivers and healthcare professionals (HCPs).

Patients with brain health conditions have evolving care needs throughout their lifespan and require support across the continuum of care: primary care, acute care, specialist services, community care, residential care and social care. Thus, the need for close cooperation between specialists from a wide variety of disciplines is strongly acknowledged by the international scientific community in view of the prospective increase in the demand for multidisciplinary services. This growingly recognised need for multi-actor and multi-level coordination is one of the key elements to be taken into account when depicting the validation scenarios for a digital health solution such as ALAMEDA, along with current service models in place, information systems' degree of interoperability, and the extent to which patients and carers participate proactively in the decision-making.

In consideration of this, the present chapter first provides a comprehensive overview of the care pathways across Europe for the three brain disorders ALAMEDA focuses on, i.e. PD, MS and stroke (the three diseases are altogether referred to as PMSS across the ALAMEDA project's documents), with a view to, first, describe the typical scenarios where the ALAMEDA suite of services and tools would be expected to be deployed and, second, provide a narrower focus on the healthcare provision system and pathways in the three pilot settings, respectively, in Italy, Greece and Romania. This way, the authors aim to illustrate hereby the main distinguishing features of care models across the EU and the relevant differences in service provision systems, referring to recent guidelines, recommendations and models for optimum care pathway where available.

Second, we will explore the extent to which shared decision-making is embedded in the diverse country-specific systems as well as the good practices, advantages and barriers to adoption. Third, we discuss the penetration of digital technologies to date, especially for what concerns the ALAMEDA research domain, i.e. patient remote monitoring and disease progression assessment. This preliminary analysis is instrumental to grasp a thorough understanding of the healthcare scenario where the ALAMEDA system is going to be tested.

Fourth, the authors provide a thorough description of the strategy adopted and activities implemented so far to implement its original participatory innovation model rooted in strong and continuous end-user engagement and cross-disciplinary fertilisation.

The data collected in the ALAMEDA pilots will support the main aims of the project, specifically:

(i) To build the ALAMEDA PMSS digital transformation and value-based impact assessment models. These will be used to attain a greater understanding of brain diseases rehabilitation treatment and address aspects that directly affect the participating actors. Active engagement of monitored persons will play a central role. The monitoring environments will span from patients' homes, medical care facilities, to outdoor surroundings.

(ii) To integrate non-disease-related factors affecting patients' quality of life into the shared decision model (SDM) for brain diseases assessment. This is done through the inclusion of, at least, 3 common data streams related to movement, cognitive functions and sleeping patterns. These will be tested via more than 15 variables related to those streams to be utilised for both disease-specific and health outcome assessment and predictive analytics. Furthermore, psychosocial, environmental and socio-economic determinants will be taken into account, too.

(iii) To develop new personalised healthcare data acquisition methods, tools and sensor prototypes that will improve and expand the landscape of monitoring possibilities during patients' daily activities, in the living environments, both indoors and outdoors. The wide outreach and applicability of the data collection tools will offer new opportunities for actionable services to be delivered to PMSS patients and their carers.

(iv) To implement new Big Data analytics and AI algorithms combined with advanced computational methods, encompassing cases of increasingly large-scale multimodal data streams that will be utilised to improve quality of life of patients with brain diseases during medical care and support.

(v) To perform ALAMEDA demonstration and small-scale validation pilots in real-world settings.

2. The Care Journey of Patients with PD, MS and Stroke

PD, MS and stroke are the three most frequent chronic neurological diseases (CNDs) that can lead to significant motor and cognitive disability: worldwide data report 2.5 million people with MS (PwMS) (Bisson *et al.*, 2019), 7.9 to 19 individuals with PD per 100,000 person-years (Muangpaisan *et al.*, 2011) and 5.5 million deaths due to stroke in 2016 (Gorelick, 2019). There are increasing rates of neurodegenerative diseases, such as PD, closely associated with the ageing population. Additionally, the prevalence and incidence of MS are increasing, especially among women, and the number of people living with stroke is estimated to increase by 27% between 2017 and 2047 in the European Union (Wafa Wolfe *et al.*, 2020), mainly because of population ageing and improved survival rates.

Despite considerable progress in symptom control, prevention of relapse and rehabilitation, unfortunately, there is still no cure for most brain disorders. Optimal care thus involves not just responding to problems expressed by patients but also adopting a proactive approach aiming to detect early warning signs that might anticipate the onset of more debilitating (and costly) problems. Personalised healthcare (PHC) recently evolved in its reinforced concept of next-PHC, which leverages 'systems biology as well as personalised, predictive, preventive, participatory and person-centred care approaches, and deploys technologies to tailor care across the health journey' (Nardini *et al.*, 2021, p. 4). In order to deliver real value to patients, a shift from a reactive care based upon disease-specific outcomes to a goal-oriented (thus, health outcome-driven) care is crucial, as is the consolidation and broader implementation of multidisciplinary and integrated care models offering the patients coordinated services across and within organisations and sectors.

Brain health is a great example given the nature of chronic brain disorders and the importance to undertake holistic efforts to offer care services beyond short-term symptomatic improvement, aiming instead at optimising functionality and quality of life. In order to translate such improvements in well-established clinical pathways and processes, it is of utmost importance to generate robust and reliable evidence to support scalability and transferability. In this regard, patient-reported outcome measures (PROMs) and patient-reported experience measures (PREMs) are essential tools to evaluate and improve healthcare results. Evaluation systems based on PROMs and PREMs may help health systems become more people-centred by providing systematic, internationally standardised information on what matters most to patients (OECD, 2019).

As highlighted by Donna Walsh, Executive Director of the European Federation of Neurological Associations, 'neurological health could be a flagship in creatively building new care pathways, paving the way for the future of healthcare in non-communicable diseases overall — whether that is in the acceleration of digital health, reconfiguring service delivery to ensure progress towards universal health coverage, developing person-alised healthcare solutions, or pushing the boundaries with breakthroughs in research and development' (EFNA, 2021, p. 7). In recent years, the emergence of ground-breaking new technologies has provided hope for further advancement towards more efficient handling of these diseases. ALAMEDA promises to support this creative process by bringing the potential of AI into the current brain health monitoring and rehabilitation/ treatment assessment practice, by employing data provided via long-term monitoring with tools (sensors and software) with minimum intervention on patient's daily life.

The following sections provide an overview of the state of play in the healthcare service provision for PMSS patients. We specifically focused our attention on the relevant dimensions that configure the current care journeys and shape the real-life scenarios for validation as well as the open issues and challenges which are important to take into account to frame the future deployment of ALAMEDA services and tools. The specific aspects examined are the extent to which care is personalised and tailored to patients' needs, multidisciplinarity, integration and coordination of care among different levels, specialities and providers, the adoption of shared decision-making models, the penetration of digital technologies and the current degree of integration and interoperability of information systems, among others.

2.1. Parkinson's disease

The global survey of neurological diseases (GBD 2016 Neurology Collaborators, 2019) revealed that the incidence and prevalence of PD have increased rapidly throughout the world. The disease affects >1.2 million people across Europe (Gustavsson *et al.*, 2011), a figure set to double by 2030 (Dorsey *et al.*, 2017). The growth can be partially explained by the ageing of the population since the incidence of PD increases with age (Bloem *et al.*, 2021). However, the risk of PD also appears to be associated with industrial chemicals and pollutants, such as pesticides (Dorsey *et al.*, 2020), metals (Weisskopf *et al.*, 2010) and solvents (Pezzoli and Cereda, 2013), which configures as the explanation for the association between larger gross national income growth rates — as a proxy for industrialisation and environmental pollution — and faster rise in the incidence of the disease (Dorsey *et al.*, 2018).

PD is a chronic, life-altering and multifaceted disease, with a highly variable presentation and disease course, and with a treatment response that can vary considerably across different individuals. The typical presentation includes a slow progression with accumulating disability for affected individuals resulting in both motor and non-motor symptoms which make the correlated personal and societal burden enormous. In daily practice, PD diagnosis is clinically based mostly on history-taking and neurological examination, while ancillary testing is reserved for people with an atypical presentation. This makes diagnosis in earlier stages particularly difficult, and delays are particularly common, e.g. when tremor is absent or in case of people with young-onset disease (Ruiz-Lopez *et al.*, 2019).

Also, the disease duration can span across decades. Because patients may live with this specific health condition for a long time, they may not be monitored regularly. Accumulating and progressing problems may be unnoticed or disregarded by the people with PD because they don't realise these are related to their condition or even due to the very smooth progression. Admission to hospital often results from a crisis occurring, with the response to management focusing on the shorter-term issue in a reactive way, and without addressing the underlying problems. This can lead to expensive, avoidable hospital admissions (NHS, 2018).

For all these reasons, complex, tailored and flexible services and multi-agency long-term provision healthcare models are required. Their administration though is often not easy to implement with the current configuration of healthcare systems and taking into account the several silos and the lack of coordination mechanisms among levels and actors. This in turn ultimately results in worse health and well-being outcomes for the people with PD, as well as higher costs for health and care services.

2.1.1. *Personalisation of care and cure*

To understand the specific challenges in current care for PD, several investigations have been conducted revealing specific unmet needs of persons with PD, their carers and HCPs involved in their care (van der Eijk *et al.*, 2011, 2012). Among others, the constraints identified include poor continuity of care and delayed detection and reactive management of symptoms. A survey by the European Parkinson's Disease Association aimed to investigate the experience of care for PD from patients' own point of view has highlighted that a shift towards more tailored healthcare, with regular and timely treatment reviews and personalised information provision, is likely to improve satisfaction with care in current healthcare pathways (Schrag *et al.*, 2018). A previous US-based study (Dorsey *et al.*, 2010) showed similar results, supporting the outcomes of the corresponding survey in Europe. Also, similar conclusions emerge from studies carried out on late-stage PD (Read *et al.*, 2019), where continuity of care for multiple symptoms and comorbidities is seen as a particular challenge given the increasing difficulty of attending medical appointments. In this context, it should be mentioned that, in the absence of continuous monitoring, the patients tend to underestimate or overestimate their status, progression or improvement by reporting only the last few days' (usually most rememberable) incidents, prior to their visits to the clinic.

There is a growing recognition that the heterogeneity of PD necessitates a highly personalised approach (Tenison *et al.*, 2020) whereby the treatment is tailored based on patients' clinical phenotype and specific symptoms. However, in which way is decision making in PD care currently personalised, i.e. tailored to the individual patient? A recent study (van den Heuvel *et al.*, 2022) has attempted to answer this question and investigate what are the main barriers hindering personalisation in care for PD. The clinicians participating in the interviews distinguished 'standard' clinical decisions from more personalised decisions. Also, different types of decisions, including medication-related decisions, lifestyle decisions and referrals to other professionals, involve different degrees of personalisation.

2.1.2. *Multidisciplinarity and integration*

Several studies have defined the ideal composition of a multidisciplinary team taking care of a person with PD as well as the configuration of the care model that would best suit the multi-faceted nature of the disease. Multidisciplinary, holistic and palliative approaches to complex needs, such as from neurologists, Parkinson's disease nurse specialists (PDNS), occupational therapists (OT), physiotherapists, speech and language therapists (SLT) and social workers (SW) are included in international and country-specific guidelines (NICE, 2017; Ferreira *et al.*, 2013).

The latest Lancet Seminar on PD (Bloem *et al.*, 2021), for instance, has highlighted the specialities and professionals deemed essential in the treatment and care of most people with PD and those competences which are required in some cases only depending on the disease manifestation, stage and individual response to treatment. Nonetheless, the inclusion of as many of these specialities in established multidisciplinary care teams might improve understanding about the complexity of PD-associated non-motor symptoms and lead to more efficient and prompt referrals to the appropriate professionals (Radder *et al.*, 2019).

Although this is not the core focus of the present chapter, it is important to acknowledge the extensive work done in the recent years on the definition of multi-actor care frameworks, which is reflected in the literature. In fact, the specific characteristics of the disease which requires optimal care involving staff from multiple (over 20 different) professional disciplines, who work in different healthcare settings, including the community, regional hospitals and specialised clinics, provide strong arguments to regard PD as an ideal model condition for other chronic neurological disorders (Bloem *et al.*, 2020). The multiple specialities involved are often referred to as 'allied health' services and providers, though several studies still report lack of PD-specific knowledge among allied health professionals and insufficient collaboration and communication among disciplines involved in PD care despite the growing evidence of its potential benefit for the patients and their quality of life (Eggers *et al.*, 2018).

There is also heterogeneity in the terminology used, with care models described most commonly as 'multidisciplinary', 'interdisciplinary' or 'integrated' (Luis-Martínez *et al.*, 2020). The majority of integrated care networks focus on care coordination involving a point of contact for PD patients and interprofessional teamwork, improving patients' education or training for specialised staff, developing various management tools and standardised processes.

A recent systematic review (Rajan *et al.*, 2020) of published integrated care models has identified several models operating across inpatient hospital care, outpatient care and community-based settings. In the *Lancet* reply to the comments on Bloem *et al.* (2020) proposing a novel network model, though, the authors acknowledge that there is still a lack of 'international agreement about relevant outcomes to evaluate the cost-effectiveness of different integrated care models, allowing for benchmarking and enabling a crucial process of learning from the differences'. This is crucial also to generate solid evidence spanning each dimension of the Quadruple Aim framework (Bodenheimer and Sinsky, 2014) and to demonstrate which models are best suited to support a shift towards value-based healthcare (Klop and Rutte, 2021).

With regard to implementation, an example of established multidisciplinary collaboration network among HCPs treating people with PD is the ParkinsonNet model in the Netherlands (Bloem and Munneke, 2014), developed with the goal of providing the best possible care and support to PD patients and their families, with an emphasis on home- and community-based care. In the same country, a further step towards enhanced care for PD patients has been marked by the design of a new model, termed PRIME Parkinson (Proactive and Integrated Management and Empowerment in Parkinson's Disease) (Tenison *et al.*, 2020) which is now being implemented in selected areas of the United Kingdom and the Netherlands with the intent of demonstrating its effectiveness (Ypinga *et al.*, 2021) in improving care while being at least cost neutral, if not generating any saving. A hub-and-spoke PD network model, based on central patient coordination and virtual integration, has been also proposed in the Lombardy region (Italy) (Albanese *et al.*, 2020).

2.1.3. *Patient involvement and shared decision-making*

Current decision-making is based on the best available scientific evidence, professional expertise and patient preferences (van den Heuvel *et al.*, 2020), although the extent to which the latter are influential on the final decisions taken is highly variable in PD due to several factors such as patient education and health literacy, lack of time, gravity of cognitive deficits, which in the context of a chronic neurodegenerative illness might pose reasonable limits to the types and amounts of information they want to know or can focus on (Zizzo *et al.*, 2017), and also the fact that HCPs are not appropriately trained for shared decision-making (SDM) (Nijhuis *et al.*, 2018). As different options for medical treatment of PD exist, SDM is getting increasingly applied in clinical decision-making. As a matter of fact, several studies have investigated how personal preferences impact treatment decisions and have resulted in confirming the importance of designing evidence-based aids (Stacey *et al.*, 2014; Bientzle *et al.*, 2020) that might inform the SDM process and help the clinicians understand patients' values and goals (Armstrong *et al.*, 2016).

On the other hand, patient involvement and SDM are most frequently documented in interventional studies concerning the decision-making process in relation to medical treatments while their application in observational studies such as ALAMEDA looks quite limited.

Also, another important aspect that should be taken into serious consideration is the differentiation between SDM and patient engagement. SDM, which is increasingly coming into focus in medical practices, features a style of communication and a set of tools that help reach a balance between medical considerations about health conditions and treatment options and an individual's preferences, goals, cultural values and beliefs. Patient engagement instead is usually referred to as the meaningful patient involvement in different aspects of care including research, care model design, guideline development, etc. In this regard, in PD healthcare research, promising participatory design efforts (Sylvie *et al.*, 2021) are being undertaken with different co-creation methods and engagement modalities, with the overall aim to steer a renovation of care models that departs from the lived experiences and care trajectories of patients and their carers.

2.1.4. *Use of technology*

PD has a relatively long prodromal period, which may allow early identification to reduce diagnostic tests for other conditions when patients simply have early symptoms of PD, as well as to reduce morbidity due to fall-related trauma. Early detection may also be essential for the development of neuroprotective therapies. In 2016, the International Parkinson and Movement Disorders Society Task Force on Technology published a summary (Espay *et al.*, 2016) of the challenges and opportunities, and lately a roadmap for the integration of technologies into PD clinical management, with a specific focus on mHealth technologies enabling the acquisition of digital outcome measures. Departing from these and the growing awareness that 'technology-based objective measures may improve the sensitivity, accuracy, reproducibility and feasibility of objectively capturing the full complexity and diversity of changes in motor and non-motor behaviors' (Espay *et al.*, 2016), a large number of experiments and studies have been conducted. Few of them, however, have rigorously investigated the feasibility and acceptability of large-scale deployment of wearable sensors, such as the Parkinson@Home study (Silva de Lima *et al.*, 2017) conducted in the US and in the Netherlands.

Overall, the potential of digital health technologies to provide objective, longitudinal and fine-grained information about the functioning of individual patients in their own home environment is generally acknowledged as is the fact that they support self-management and improve communication between the patients and the HCPs. It is worth mentioning that despite the fact that wearables are not as accurate as clinical/medical devices within the premises of a clinic, the continuous monitoring of patients leading to accumulation of large number of objective measurements ('big data') will provide a complementary source of information that can span large periods of time of monitoring the real-life conditions of the patients. The possibility to depict digital health pathways (Klucken *et al.*, 2018) for people with PD largely depends on the deployment of those technologies, coupled with the improved connectivity enabled by electronic health records and digital patient management platforms as well as the disruptive introduction of big data research, which is promising to improve knowledge on disease mechanisms, diagnostic and therapeutic strategies. This will in turn allow the shift from a triple to a quadruple decision-making model for PD, where scientific evidence, professional expertise and patient preferences are integrated with big data approaches, thus setting the basis for a paradigmatic advance in precision medicine (van den Heuvel *et al.*, 2020), which is still far from being applicable in PD as of this writing. Challenges include, among others, difficulty identifying, as well as lack of consensus on, digital outcomes, quality of data, low digital and health literacy in vulnerable population groups, interoperability and device compatibility, as well as lack of evidence-supported incentives for payers which translate into missing reimbursement schemes, thus hindering innovation and deployment.

A specific area demanding further development is indeed patient remote monitoring, which is the ALAMEDA research core domain. van Halteren *et al.* (2021) define proactive monitoring as the 'timely detection of the first changes in signs or symptoms, allowing for pre-emptive interventions to prevent further worsening of problems and to avoid complications that might lead to emergency department visits, hospital admission and use of unnecessary resources'. In this sense, the authors regard early detection of signs and symptoms through proactive monitoring as one of the five core elements needed to achieve optimal personalised care management, along with care coordination, patient navigation, information provision and process monitoring. All these elements can be promisingly supported by digital technologies, and their use is spreading widely although with several differences in technological maturity.

In fact, while several devices and solutions for detection and monitoring of motor symptoms have reached the highest level of development and have been approved by regulatory agencies in the EU and USA for routine clinical practice (e.g. for the remote monitoring of axial motor symptoms, bradykinesia and tremor) (Luis-Martínez *et al.*, 2020), with regard to non-motor clinical manifestations (van Wamelen *et al.*, 2021), fewer studies have looked into the deployment of wearable and remote technology for their measurement and monitoring, for which demonstration of clinical utility and user acceptance is inherently more complex.

2.2. *Multiple sclerosis*

MS is an inflammatory disorder of the central nervous system (CNS) and one of the world's most common neurological conditions. In many countries, it is the leading cause of non-traumatic disability in young adults and symptoms include vision problems, spasticity, weakness, ataxia, bladder and bowel dysfunctions, fatigue, pain syndromes, tremors, vertigo, cognitive impairment and mood disorders (Kes *et al.*, 2013).

MS occurs when the immune system attacks the protective layer around healthy nerve cells, causing damage to the pathways that transmit signals throughout the brain and body. It is classified by disease stage and permanence of symptoms.

Most MS cases begin as Clinically Isolated Syndromes and then manifest as either relapsing-remitting MS (RRMS), which features alternating periods of disease activity and remission, or primary progressive MS (PPMS), which has increasing disease activity without periods of remission. After years or decades, most RRMS cases will advance to Secondary Progressive MS (SPMS), which presents similarly to PPMS (Montalban *et al.*, 2018) (Figure 1). Conversion from RRMS to SPMS

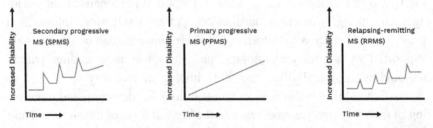

Figure 1.   Most common clinical courses of MS (Adapted from Lublin and Reingold, 1996).

is considered a key determinant of long-term disease prognosis and, in addition to augmented uncertainty and progressively increasing disease severity, it brings relevant psychosocial problems for patients and caregivers (Solari *et al.*, 2019).

Currently, MS diagnosis is the combined outcome of clinical presentation with conventional laboratory tests and imaging (and, in some cases, additional tests to reject alternative possible disorders).

While there is currently no cure for MS, the condition can be managed through specialised healthcare support, starting with early diagnosis. Once the patient has been diagnosed, MS care focuses on reducing progression with disease-modifying drugs (DMDs), symptom management and rehabilitation to maintain quality of life and neurological function.

The unpredictability of MS along with the young average age at onset (between 20 and 40 years) means that it could disrupt personal development, social participation and productivity as people are affected during the formative years of their life, when they may be looking to complete their education, establish a career or start a family. Thus, the disease generates a direct and indirect impact on the economy, employment, and health and social care systems (Kobelt *et al.*, 2017). Furthermore, MS places a unique burden on women since females are twice as likely to have MS than men globally, with some countries reporting a much higher ratio up to 4:1, as shown by the findings of the open-source global compendium of data compiled by the Multiple Sclerosis International Federation (MSIF) between 2019 and 2020 (Walton *et al.*, 2020).

2.2.1. *Personalisation of care and cure*

In recent years, treatment and care for MS have become increasingly multifaceted requiring multidisciplinary input and regular monitoring, with adaptable and person-centred approaches.

With regard to disease management and, ultimately, cure, experts agree that the application of precision medicine will be a necessary next step in MS future research as the heterogeneity in disease course, wide variety of clinical expressions as well as treatment response and correlated risks demonstrates that there are a number of critical decision points (i.e. risk detection, diagnosis, prognosis, treatment response and disease progression) in MS management that would benefit from such an approach leveraging validated predictors/biomarkers (Chitnis and Prat, 2020).

Coordinated collection and sharing of data, development of predictive models and their progressive evaluation in the care of individual patients will be an essential and challenging part of this in the years to come. Also, to ensure that the promises of personalised medicine for MS are realised, researchers must engage with PwMS's lived experiences, to develop and adapt truly personalised approaches (Henschke *et al.*, 2021).

Similarly, with regard to the design and provision of personalised rehabilitation plans and services, important steps are being taken in terms of their customisation and tailoring (Hvid *et al.*, 2021) to the domains and needs that are most meaningful to patients (Brichetto and Zaratin, 2020) as well as in progressing towards accurate prediction of their effectiveness (Kanzler *et al.*, 2022). For MS as well as for other neurological conditions, a critical aspect towards the personalisation, especially related to accurate prediction and effectiveness, is the large size of accumulated information for each patient (or alternatively for groups of patients that are tightly intercorrelated in terms of the disease phenotype and their response to it), i.e. data gathered over long periods of time.

2.2.2. *Multidisciplinarity and integration*

Similarly to other neurological, complex and chronic conditions, monitoring and management of the diverse MS symptoms and disease-modifying therapy (DMT) side effects as well as potential comorbidities (Marrie, 2017) across the patient's life course require the specialist neurologist to draw on expertise from a wide range of disciplines across health and social care.

However, it has been proven difficult to provide high-quality interdisciplinary care, namely due to existing information management silos, lack of communication between the health and social care systems, as well as due to resource shortage, which translates into low numbers of specialists and large caseloads. All of these pose considerable barriers to interdisciplinary working and harm the capacity of the healthcare systems to provide personalised care and foster patient engagement and education.

There is a consolidated awareness and support from the scientific literature and the international MS community that a multidisciplinary approach integrating patients' care (diagnosis, treatment, monitoring and follow-up) and rehabilitation activities (including neuropsychological and social support) would enhance the efficacy of care and provide better overall patient satisfaction (Vermersch *et al.*, 2016). On this basis and departing from the learnings accumulated in other relative disease domains, a conceptual model setting the minimum components that the ideal MS Care Unit should include has been designed, with the MS neurologist and MS specialist nurse occupying the central role in the management of all patients with MS (Soelberg Sorensen *et al.*, 2019).

Recent reports have highlighted that there are still large differences among countries in terms of quality of care, access at MS clinics for regular monitoring and interdisciplinary collaboration and coordination, which makes it likely that the task of coordinating care falls to the person with MS and her/his caregivers, thus contributing to the rise of health inequalities which have been amplified by the COVID-19 pandemic (Di Luca *et al.*, 2020). In this regard, a cross-sectional online survey conducted by FISM researchers in Italy showed that patients with MS reported experiencing worse self-reported health status and difficulty to access care, support and rehabilitation services during the country-wide lockdown, although detrimental impacts in different care domains have been differently perceived by people with earlier diagnosis and patients with more severe and advanced disease manifestations (Manacorda *et al.*, 2021).

Moreover, sub-optimal healthcare services available to patients with MS usually lead to a greater use of informal care (Kanavos *et al.*, 2016) (which was a trend confirmed and exacerbated during the pandemic) and, consequently, a heavier burden on personal and family economy. With a view to guiding future investments in reforming MS management, some studies (Moral Torres *et al.*, 2020) have estimated the potential social value and economic savings which could be pursued by making MS healthcare services more accessible and integrated.

2.2.3. *Patient involvement and shared decision-making*

The SDM model (Elwyn *et al.*, 2012) has been shown to facilitate adherence to MS treatment by taking patient values and preferences into consideration (Ben-Zacharia *et al.*, 2018; Colligan *et al.*, 2017; Eskyte *et al.*, 2019). Among the relevant barriers for its effective use to promote truly patient-centred care, skill development programs for HCPs are still insufficient or lacking. In the MS care field, shared decision making is more broadly established as a practice in the early stages of RRMS while its adoption shows a decline as disease severity increases (Brown *et al.*, 2018). A recent mixed-method study (Péloquin *et al.*, 2021) showed that for neurologists the greatest educational needs relate to managing side effects and providing care aligned with patients' personal goals and quality of life.

Within the realm of shared decision-making theoretical models, advance care planning (ACP) is a process that 'enables individuals who have decisional capacity to identify their values, to reflect upon the meanings and consequences of serious illness scenarios, to define goals and preferences for future medical treatment and care, and to discuss these with family and HCPs' (Rietjens *et al.*, 2017). As it aims to involve doctors, patients and families on decision-making based on an anticipated deterioration in the health status of a patient, thus including plans for the time the patients will eventually lose decisional capacity, ACP is indeed an area where the inclusion of appropriate training in medical education is of crucial importance. Also, central to the adoption of patient education and HCP training interventions for ACP in MS is the need to generate robust evidence on its benefits, which is the major goal of the ongoing ConCureMS study supported by the Italian MS Society (AISM) Foundation (De Panfilis *et al.*, 2021).

Overall, we have increasing access to methods and devices fostering patient participation in maintenance of health, pursuit of tailored and timely treatment, involvement in research and contribution to priority setting. A recent meta-synthesis of people's experiences of living with MS (Desborough *et al.*, 2020) identified five key themes that describe the most important areas where these advances can generate implications for patients: (1) the quest for knowledge, expertise and understanding,

(2) uncertain trajectories, (3) loss of valued roles and activities, and the threat of a changing identity, (4) managing fatigue and its impacts on life and relationships, and (5) adapting to life with MS. In all these areas, pros, cons, limiting factors and enablers of patient engagement in MS research and healthcare must be thoroughly considered in order to maximise benefits and avoid unintended effects, such as increased uncertainty or overwhelming information excess (Henschke *et al.*, 2021).

2.2.4. *Use of technology*

Similarly to the PD case, in the present section, we concentrate, in particular, on the promise held by the progressively growing evidence supporting the use of technological aids and advanced data collection, analysis and interpretation methods and tools in the area of disease progression monitoring, assessment, response to treatment and, ultimately, outcome prediction as this is the focus of ALAMEDA.

Despite the significant role of managing and reducing relapses in the care of MS patients, many go unreported. According to a survey in the UK, one in two PwMS fail to report a relapse (Duddy *et al.*, 2014), highlighting the importance of close monitoring. A patient's well-being, relapses and symptoms are reviewed during their annual or six-monthly neurology consultation, but due to the long period of time between outpatient visits, patients often tend to attach more relevance to relatively more recent events, resulting in a biased and, to a certain extent, limited reporting of symptoms.

Remote patient monitoring tools may allow more continuous and objective monitoring, either via passive sensing or allowing patients to record symptoms in a standardised format on a day-to-day basis.

Digital therapeutics, wearable technology and self-management apps also play an essential role in the empowerment of patients by increasing awareness about their health and their ability to manage their own condition (Brichetto *et al.*, 2019). Connecting caregivers and patients through such tools in an integrated and constructive manner will also ameliorate shared decision making and can improve a patient's commitment to therapy and their satisfaction, which in turn translates into better health outcomes. Furthermore, the exploitation of novel technologies, such as virtual reality (VR) and Exergame, are suggested as a supplement to the rehabilitation therapy of MS patients (Trombini *et al.*, 2021) in the cutting-edge frontier of Internet of Medical Things (IoMT) research.

Increasing digitalisation and the availability of easy-to-use devices and technology also enable HCPs to use a new class of digital biomarkers (Dillenseger *et al.*, 2021) to explain, influence and/or predict health-related outcomes. The technology and devices from which these digital biomarkers stem are quite broad, and range from wearables that collect patients' activity during digitalised functional tests (e.g. the Multiple Sclerosis Performance Test, dual-tasking performance and speech) to digitalised diagnostic procedures (e.g. optical coherence tomography) and software-supported magnetic resonance imaging evaluation. The greater the progress in the research in this field, and the more and larger the real-world data studies (Mowry *et al.*, 2020) conducted, the closer the realisation of the full potential of digital biomarkers as the cornerstone in the path towards real-life data acquisition, the closer the patient monitoring and thus the larger the available datasets essential for precision medicine.

Digital biomarkers are also an important component of the so-called digital twins (Voigt *et al.*, 2021), a promising technological innovation potentially deployable for several long-term complex diseases such as MS. A digital twin in healthcare is a virtual copy of a patient that exactly matches that patient's characteristics and attributes, thus mirroring the patient, and allowing for simulation and treatment response prediction.

Challenges around infrastructure, evidence generation, privacy and security issues, consistent data collection and workflow, and HCPs' lack of trust remain along with the need for legislative actions, standards and evidence-based guidelines based upon clinical validation studies in real-world environments.

2.3. Stroke

The third brain disease which ALAMEDA concentrates upon is the stroke. Ischemic strokes make up about 80% of all strokes (Aguilar, 2015). Just as a heart attack occurs when there is insufficient blood flow to the heart, an ischemic stroke (sometimes called a 'brain attack') occurs when there is a sudden interruption in blood flow to one or more regions of the brain, which represents the second most common cause of death worldwide (WHO, 2020) and a leading cause of adult physical disability (Murray *et al.*, 2012). As for other neurological conditions, an important contributing factor to this is that the number of older persons in Europe is rising, with a projected increase of 35% between 2017 and 2050 (United Nations, 2017).

A joint report released by the Stroke Alliance for Europe (SAFE) and the University of Oxford estimates the costs of stroke will increase from €60 billion in 2017 (Luengo-Fernandez *et al.*, 2020) to €86 billion in 2040, with the 2017 overall costs including the costs for direct healthcare provision, the costs of social care services, the estimated economic burden of informal and unpaid care provided by relatives and informal caregivers, and the loss of productivity caused by deaths and disability (SAFE & University of Oxford, 2020).

Moreover, in the last two years, it has become strikingly evident that individuals with acquired brain injury such as stroke may be particularly vulnerable to changes in healthcare utilisation because of ongoing healthcare needs such as the extraordinary disruption in services prompted by the COVID-19 pandemic (Kim *et al.*, 2021), testified by the decreased number of admissions for fear of contagion as reported in many countries (Zhao *et al.*, 2020).

Significant progress has been made in the last decades to balance the 'relative disequilibrium' (O'Neill *et al.*, 2008) in acute event treatment, i.e. the 'front end of stroke' care, and progressively acknowledge the equal importance of post-acute care involving secondary prevention, chronic disease management and rehabilitation, which involve those steps of the stroke care journey ALAMEDA mostly aspires to contribute to enhance (see Figure 2).

The focus of post-acute care is on reducing mortality, maximising recovery and preventing recurrent stroke and cardiovascular events. In well-developed countries, post-acute stroke outcome has been steadily improving in recent years thanks to intense and more tailored

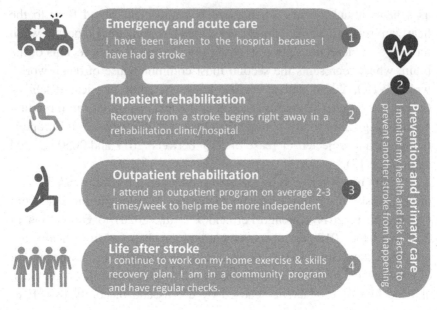

Figure 2.   The stroke patient's journey.

rehabilitation programmes and coupled pharmacological and non-pharmacological secondary prevention interventions (Bonkhoff and Grefkes, 2021).

Specifically, rehabilitation refers to the entire process of care after brain injury and an 'active change by which a person who has become disabled acquires the knowledge and skills needed for optimum physical, psychological and social function' (British Society of Rehabilitation Medicine, 2003).

As highlighted by the authors of a European Stroke Organisation's blog at the end of March 2020 'before the pandemic, during and after, stroke remains'. Indeed, several organisations have warned about the direct and indirect effects of COVID-19 pressure on healthcare systems, which has negatively affected the timeliness and quality of care provided to patients who have suffered from a stroke and high-level panels of experts have formulated recommendations to mitigate those effects (Venketasubramanian et al., 2021).

2.3.1. *Personalisation of care and cure*

Currently, personalised aspects of prevention of stroke include tailoring interventions based on global risk, the utilisation of individualised management plans within a model of organised care, and patient education (Kim *et al.*, 2015).

However, stroke is regarded as a suitable candidate for precision medicine which holds the promise of true personalisation for all phases of stroke care — prevention, acute treatment and rehabilitation (Herrgårdh *et al.*, 2021), in order to tackle the stochastic response of people who suffered a stroke due to their treatment and create specific patient-oriented management. To achieve this goal, efforts to collect, value and synthesise the wealth of data collected in clinical trials and routine care are indispensable (Hinman *et al.*, 2017).

2.3.2. *Multidisciplinarity and integration*

Very notable progress has been made in the treatment and management of acute and in-patient post-acute stroke across Europe with the establishment and consolidation of stroke care units. Evidence of the effectiveness of stroke unit care and the benefits of thrombolysis have transformed treatment for people after stroke.

In most countries, inpatient stroke rehabilitation is underpinned by evidence-based National Clinical Guidelines (see, e.g. Jauch *et al.*, 2013) and relies on a coordinated team approach to planning, delivering and evaluating care. The evidence supporting its effectiveness has been collated in several systematic reviews published since 2000.

However, it has been observed that with regard to early support discharge (ESD) and long-term rehabilitation, the degree of integration is varied and many stroke survivors still experience a poor transition from hospital to home, insufficient information provision and inefficient coordination and follow-up. For instance, there are still considerable differences across regions and countries in the way in-patient and ESD or community-based stroke teams work collaboratively to ensure that the patient and carer are fully informed of what services (if any) are provided post-discharge as well as the extent to which allied rehabilitation actors and service providers are informed about patients' needs and able to provide the required aid effectively and in a timely manner.

It emerges that the improvements achieved in acute treatment and inpatient management now need to be matched by increasing focus on longer-term support (Clarke and Forster, 2015).

2.3.3. Patient involvement and shared decision-making

SDM is relevant for therapeutic and healthcare choices throughout stroke care, from thrombolysis to goals of care, diagnostic assessments, rehabilitation strategies and secondary stroke prevention (Armstrong, 2017). Recent studies have investigated the barriers and facilitators for SDM with patients with stroke (Voogdt-Pruis *et al.*, 2019). In fact, stroke can limit patients' understanding of complex information about care options and their anticipated outcomes, consequently impeding patient participation in the decision-making process (Suleman and Kim, 2015). Cognitive problems in patients with stroke (such as memory problems, a poor understanding of the condition or the inability to judge adequately) as well as communication problems such as aphasia or dysarthria could also hinder the SDM process. Furthermore, lack of HCPs' training and resources represents a hindering factor also in this case. Nonetheless, embedding the timely investigation of patients' preferences in the care process — before starting treatment discussions and with the involvement of a multidisciplinary group of professionals as well as relatives and caregivers — is considered both feasible and recommendable.

Two basic principles influence approaches to patient post-acute treatment and rehabilitation. The first is that the adult CNS is adaptive, or plastic, and has some capacity to reorganise itself to recover degraded cognitive and motor functions. The second principle is that progressive, skilled motor practice is essential for continued gains at any time after stroke onset via physical rehabilitation. For these, both cognitive and physical rehabilitation are crucial for stroke survivors. However, the application of SDM in follow-up monitoring and rehabilitation plans is neither widespread nor documented. Most recent publications on SDM in stroke care mostly focus on oral anticoagulation for stroke prevention in atrial fibrillation (see, e.g. Ferguson and Hendriks, 2017), which is also the domain where some established decision aids (DAs) are being utilised, while less research exists for other decisions relating to stroke and especially for post-acute treatment, follow up and rehabilitation.

2.3.4. *Use of technology*

A trend like the one we are witnessing in several other chronic disease domains is characterising stroke healthcare: as cost pressures increase and healthcare networks become increasingly consolidated, pressure is growing to leverage digital health solutions to create more affordable, high-quality and convenient (from the patient's perspective) stroke healthcare (Schwamm *et al.*, 2017). In stroke care, the advantages brought about by the adoption of digital technologies span across the full range of phases of the patient journey. As ineffective systems of care may be a factor associated with worse stroke outcomes and, therefore, they are an important area of focus (Adeoye *et al.*, 2019), digital technologies undoubtedly represent part of the answer to address such inefficiencies.

AI-based prediction approaches hold several advantages in the field of post-stroke recovery especially for their potential capacity to explain non-linear relationships and interactions (Bonkhoff and Grefkes, 2021), not easily conceived even by experts in the field. The availability of predictions may help HCPs, caregivers and patients to be informed about what to expect in the future and to plan accordingly, in a timely manner. Outcome models could also target the prediction of response to specific therapies, such as non-invasive brain stimulation (Ovadia-Caro *et al.*, 2019).

On the other hand, mHealth technology provides a novel way to promote adherence to home exercise programmes post stroke (Grau-Pellicer *et al.*, 2020). Telerehabilitation (either by phone, via videoconferencing software or through dedicated apps) (Iodice *et al.*, 2021) and assistive technologies (Harris and Sthapit, 2016) allowing patients to perform rehabilitation routines themselves have demonstrated to provide an extensive benefit for stroke recovery. During circumstances such as the COVID-19 pandemic, telerehabilitation can be critically useful to limit in-person consultation making optimal secondary prevention and rehabilitation feasible at home, minimise costly human intervention, and help reduce the impact of stroke on the economy and healthcare system. Also, decision support aids such as algorithm-based apps for OT are becoming increasingly diffused (Hancock *et al.*, 2019) as they help guide therapy choices based on best research evidence for the movement impairments the patients experience.

3. From Care Journeys to ALAMEDA Validation Scenarios

3.1. *The Greek pilot scenario*

The Greek healthcare organisation involved in the ALAMEDA pilot testing is the Special Outpatient Clinic of Parkinson's Disease and Related Movement Disorders. This clinic aims to diagnose and treat patients with either PD or other movement disorders (including tremors, dystonia and atypical parkinsonian syndromes). The outpatient Clinic of Parkinson's Disease and related Movement Disorders belongs to the First Department of Neurology of the National and Kapodistrian University of Athens (NKUA) Medical School. The Clinic is located centrally in Athens, within the facilities of Aiginiteio Hospital. In this Clinic, patients are usually self-referred, but occasionally referrals from other colleagues also occur. The patients are predominantly from Athens or the Attica area, but many of them are also from other Greek regions. PD patients in need of admission are admitted to a speciality ward of Aiginiteio Hospital dedicated to patients with neurodegenerative disorders.

The outpatient Clinic is staffed by neurologists who are either university professors or hospital staff, while there are also collaborating neurologists assisting. The Chief Nurse has a specialisation in CNDs and the management of their symptoms and burden. The multidisciplinary team also includes a collaborating psychologist, a neuropsychologist (university professor), a nutritionist, a social worker and a psychiatrist assisting in the Clinic. An estimated 700 patients with PD per year are treated in the Clinic: they are attended and monitored by two specialised neurology professors who visit 45 patients every month on average. After diagnosis, follow-up visits are scheduled every 6 or 12 months and last approximately half an hour although the neurologists report that the first visits in the early follow-up phase can take considerably longer. This category, i.e. recently diagnosed and in need of early assessment and follow-up, groups the highest number of patients attended in the Clinic, although several patients in advanced stages of the disease with both motor and non-motor fluctuations are also attended to.

Clinical data are collected, recorded and stored in the Clinic database. Specifically, a narrative medical history is kept for each patient, along with the results of his/her examinations, as well as the diagnostic tests, the diagnosis and the disease management plan. Depending on the individual needs, specific tests are administered to the patients, and they are recorded too, e.g. the Mini-Mental State Examination (MMSE), or the Montreal Cognitive Assessment (MoCA), the Global Deterioration Scale (GDS), Unified Parkinson's Disease Rating Scale UPDRS-III and -IV if necessary.

Currently, these data are accessible only to the team of each University Professor who is in charge of specific patients. There is no automatic sharing system in place as yet at the time of writing between the Clinic and external allied healthcare providers eventually involved in the care plan nor with the GPs. External HCPs, such as physiatrists, speech therapists, etc., receive a written report with a specific request to attend to the patient. On the other hand, patients and their caregivers do not have direct access to the clinical records: they can obtain formal reports of their condition that are issued upon request, usually for insurance purposes.

PROMs and PREMs are not collected on a routine basis, though the Clinic participates in clinical research studies. Where relevant, data on quality of life are gathered by administering the Parkinson's Disease Questionnaire (PDQ-8 or PDQ-39). Such information is also to be collected as part of the ALAMEDA study. Altogether, these experiments represent promising steps forward and are expected to pave the way to a more systematic and structured engagement of patients in care planning and improving healthcare service provision, which is also the goal pursued by a recently established local patient society, already informed about ALAMEDA and involved in our actions via the Local Community Group established in the context of the project's patient engagement plan (see Section 4).

Remote monitoring is not established as a routine healthcare practice. The clinic is participating in a study experimenting a medical device for continuous monitoring of movement disorders, called PD Monitor.[1] This is applied for a period of three consecutive days approximately over the period of one month and can be repeated. The system has five recording sites (limb and waist) and aims to capture the on-and-off states in patients with motor complications.

3.2. The Italian pilot scenario

The Italian Multiple Sclerosis Foundation (FISM) is the leading funding and research organisation in the field of MS in Italy. The intramural research areas include rehabilitation and public health, in particular through smart, robotic and immersive devices both for monitoring and for rehabilitation assistance in the clinical, home and work setting.

FISM is the research branch of the AISM which addresses several aspects of MS, through advocating for the rights of PwMS and providing services such as information desks, social support, well-being activities and rehabilitation management.

AISM rehabilitation centres are out-patient structures aimed at improving PwMS's quality of life through the recovery and maintenance of residual functions and an active participation in social life. They collaborate with hospitals and territorial services, both receiving patients who received a diagnosis of MS in order to schedule a rehabilitative plan and referring PwMS for specialist visits.

In the AISM rehabilitation services, a global rehabilitation interdisciplinary approach is proposed: different professional figures (physiatrists, physiotherapists, speech therapists, nurses, OT, SW or other figures depending on the different centres) take care of the global management of the person with MS through a common decision-making process and the sharing of objectives.

Services offered include a first interdisciplinary visit (physiatrists, psychologist, social worker and nurse), specialist medical activities (e.g. orthopaedic or swallowing visits, instrumental exams for motor or bladder deficit, acupuncture, etc.), individual or group rehabilitation, speech therapy, psychological support and diet prescription.

---

[1] https://www.pdneurotechnology.com/pd-monitor-solution/product/.

All activities are managed through continuous experts' integration and coordination, with internal weekly scheduled meetings in order to discuss about patients' clinical aspects.

The AISM Centre participating in the ALAMEDA pilot activities is based in the city of Genova (Liguria Region, Italy). More than 1,200 PwMS receive a visit and rehabilitative treatment every year (either in the centre or at home).

The AISM Rehabilitation Centre does not provide neurological visits, which are in the responsibility of hospitals and MS centres connected with AISM. At the AISM Rehabilitation Centre, the rehabilitative programme is set by physiatrists and concerted with the multidisciplinary team described above.

At the centre, each psychiatrist visits about 40 patients every month. Visits are scheduled every 6 months approximately and their duration can vary from one hour (follow-up visits) to three hours (first visit).

Neurological status, functional domains status through clinician-assessed outcomes (CAOs), patient-reported outcomes (PROs) and performance measures (PMs) are the clinical areas for which data are collected on a routine basis. Data are stored in a central database that can be accessed by the healthcare professional of the AISM. Similarly to the Greek scenario, there is no systematic data-sharing system in place connecting the AISM database and hospital or MS specialistic centre databases. In general, data are shared in paper format with the neurologist of the MS centres that are linked with the AISM rehabilitation centres to manage the care process. Moreover, additional information (paper format) can be shared with allied specialists depending on the need.

A personalised care and rehabilitation plan is shared with the patient and his/her carers. Taking into account the patients' goals and recommendations by the specialist, the rehabilitation programme is set, and the results are communicated at the end.

Clinical outcomes (CAOs, PROs and PMs) are collected before and after each rehabilitative treatment by the therapists of the centre.

Moreover, a study is currently ongoing in order to create a large dataset of outcomes in PwMS (PROMOPROMS) (Brichetto *et al.*, 2020). Personal (i.e. years of education), clinical (i.e. number of relapses in the last 4 months) and biometric (i.e. height and weight) data, PROs and CAOs related to the most relevant domains for MS (i.e. mobility, fatigue, cognitive performances, emotional status, bladder continence, quality of life), were acquired every 4 months since 2014. Up until now, about 8,000 evaluations from more than 1,000 patients have been collected.

Following the several initiatives in place that are contributing to demonstrate the benefits of active and effective patient engagement in healthcare management and decision-making, a patient engagement initiative has been put in place from the healthcare authorities of Liguria Region (namely, ALISA, the regional company in charge of the planning and control function of health and social services). The overall aim is to personalise and humanise health services and place the person with the disease (with his/her feelings, knowledge and beliefs) at the centre of care, thus consolidating an initiative which is highly relevant to connect with for ALAMEDA research and its potential scaling up at the regional level.

3.3. *The Romanian pilot scenario*

The University Emergency Hospital Bucharest (SUUB) is one of the largest hospitals in Romania. The Neurology Department participating in the ALAMEDA study includes neurologists, researchers, neuropsychologists and support staff dedicated to the highest quality of patient care using the most advanced technologies, integrated treatments, clinical research and multidisciplinary, integrated patient care.

In particular, the stroke pilot is being run by the clinical staff and researchers working at the emergency department thus dealing mostly with patients with acute stroke, the most frequent pathology being ischemic stroke.

After patients are treated at the emergency unit, they are guided through the first phase of their rehabilitation journey via in-patient therapy and recommendations of out-patient programmes after discharge. Towards this aim, the emergency team collaborates closely with a physiotherapist and with a physical therapist in order to help the stroke patient with the transition from the acute phase of stroke towards the rehabilitation phase.

With regard to the type of the emergency assistance provided, it is not possible to provide an average number of outpatient visits performed by each neurologist as follow-up consultations are not performed by this unit. After discharge, the patient is referred to a neurologist in an outpatient service to receive appropriate follow-up. Only in some cases is a follow-up visit after discharge scheduled, depending on what the patient needs, e.g. for patients with carotid stenting, follow-up is scheduled at 3, 6, 9 and 12 months and, also, for patients with suspected neurocognitive disorders, at 3 months.

During the in-hospital stay, the journey to rehabilitation begins with the support of a team made of doctors, nurses, a physiotherapist and a physical therapist. An exercise programme is established and slowly the patient starts to practise. At discharge, the patient and the caregivers are given all the results from medical examinations as well as further recommendations. The patient is instructed to follow the physical exercises recommended by the physical therapist and is referred to a rehabilitation clinic.

All clinical exams and all medical data are recorded in the digital system used by SUUB during visits and are available to the HCPs of the department in order to compare data regarding a patient's evolution. It is not shared nor connected to other healthcare information systems in other hospitals or regions. In SUUB, only doctors have access to patients' files: the other healthcare providers, e.g. nurses, physiotherapists and physical therapists, may also have access. External professionals they collaborate with must request access.

Patients receive all the results from their examinations as well as a written report on the disease status, evolution and recommendations. If necessary, the patient must sign an informed consent to allow to provide the same data to the caregiver.

To date, at SUUB there is no system in place to collect data related to PROMs and/or PREMs nor remote monitoring systems at home.

To the best knowledge of SUUB professionals, currently there is no systematic local or regional programme to engage the patients, collect data from patients' post-stroke experience and outcomes, and plan improvements in the rehabilitation and post-stroke care service provision.

4. Engagement of the End Users in the R&I Process

Despite the huge progress made and the impetus given by COVID-19 to countries to accelerate the adoption of digital health, it is largely acknowledged that challenges with the adoption, scale and spread of health innovations still represent significant gaps in the evidence-to-practice cycle (Bird *et al.*, 2021). In the health innovation design process, a lack of attention paid to the needs of end-users, and subsequent tailoring of innovations to meet these needs, is deemed as one of the most likely reasons for the failed adoption of many promising innovations. Thus, in the recent years, digital health developers and providers have been broadly exploring the best ways to keep the human element at front and centre of the digital health innovation process.

Furthermore, the engagement of end users unavoidably acquires centrality regardless of the sector, as long as the innovation community is consistently shifting from a *product design* to a *service design* approach. When a technology (tool) includes a clearly stated, meaningful value proposition (Shaw *et al.*, 2018) for all users who must interact with the technology or the information it generates, the newly introduced technology can be used as a trigger for establishing new routines involved in providing care, and ultimately a re-configured service or even an improved treatment or care pathway.

This has led to a progressive acknowledgement of the primary importance attached to end users' engagement, as recently recognised also in guidance documents made available by health authorities, payers and HTA agencies in order to support innovators in understanding what the health systems and providers are looking for when buying digital and data-driven technology for use in health and care, so that these principles of good practice can be built into the strategy and product development 'by design'. An example is provided by the recently updated UK 'Code of Conduct for Data-Driven Health and Care Technologies' which explicitly refers to end users' engagement as follows: 'One of the best practical ways of getting to a clear value proposition is to research and define user needs thoroughly, and then involve users as much as possible in the whole life cycle of the product, through discovery, design, change and post-release review. Understanding the people and their specific needs will help with uptake and adoption of the technology or innovation being built, as well as clearly showing a commissioner or buyer the problem being solved' (UK Government Department of Health, 2021).

Furthermore, the approval of Regulation 2282/2021 (HTA Regulation) (European Commission, 2021) has marked a renewed acknowledgement of patient engagement centrality. Within its new legislation frame, which entails a three-year transition period towards effective application as of 2025, Member States will have a new permanent framework for a European Cooperation on HTA and common rules to perform HTA jointly at the European level. The HTA Regulation also establishes quality standards for the joint work: among them, it requires the systematic and timely participation of patient experts in the procedures of the new Cooperation, especially in the main activities, such as Joint Scientific Consultations and Joint Clinical Assessments.

In ALAMEDA, the primary end users are identified as follows:

Patients with Parkinson's disease, multiple sclerosis and stroke (PMSS): They will benefit from the individual personalised care based on AI decision-making models that may be tuned to cover various aspects of brain diseases and a variety of medical care models, as well as methods to calibrate such models for individuals. Advanced data analytics and AI systems are being deployed in order to: (i) continuously monitor their health status and overall cognitive capacity; (ii) evaluate outcomes that matter to patients, such as fatigue, psychosocial status, anxiety and depression, quality of life, and satisfaction with the technology and telehealthcare.

Healthcare professionals: The developed AI methods will be able to integrate and handle efficiently heterogeneous datasets and datasets with missing values (incomplete data). Different patients and outcomes will be monitored and recorded at different frequencies mainly due to the differences in their health status and the symptoms, enabling clinicians to design personalised monitoring plans. Further, medical doctors will be provided with bias-free information concerning the patients' life and disease-related incidents, as inferred by the AI and monitoring process between the on-site clinical visits. Relapses have a major influence on clinicians' treatment decisions for patients with PMSS, therefore, equipping clinicians with advanced tools for on-time prediction of relapse is of utmost importance to identify the most appropriate treatment, ensuring effective care for these patients over time. Monitoring motor function and sleep characteristics has the potential to predict the course of the disease, in particular, the prediction of relapse or worsening that is fundamental for improving drugs and rehabilitative treatments' efficacy, resulting in a better care and quality of life for the people affected by PMSS. For example, there are pointers in the PD case where sleep and motor incidents and their properties may help the clinical doctors towards decisions concerning whether more drastic actions apart from drug administration should take place, early enough, before the quality of the patient's life is severely downgraded.

Caregivers: The role of caregiving has a large socio-emotional impact that cannot be ignored. As this impact grows, families are looking for innovative solutions to help them balance the needs of patients with the demands of caregiving. There is encouraging and progressively increasing engagement of caregivers and their associations and networks in digital health and health innovation. A recent survey carried out on more than 700 caregivers in the US (Massachusetts eHealth Institute, 2017) found that the majority considered the opportunity to use digital health solutions 'very appealing'. This included technology that provides 'access to test results and other medical records in one place'; 'reliable information about the needs and conditions of patients'; and 'tools to communicate directly with doctors and other care providers and coordinators'. Digital health technology can indeed help address the adverse health complications that caregivers face by, e.g. building communities for peer-to-peer interaction and support, assisting in managing everyday tasks and improving the ability of caregivers to monitor health and medications. Specifically, ALAMEDA intends to contribute to the latter objective by providing a comprehensive, multi-sensor monitoring solution for individuals with brain disorders, deploying a great variety of sensors to monitor their physiological status, overall health and lifestyle aspects. The heterogeneous sensor data will be integrated in an intelligent manner, resulting in a comprehensive picture of the person's current status and its evolution over time, allowing the HCPs to determine the best care approach in each case. Each sensing modality will be analysed separately, and their results will be integrated in a semantically meaningful manner, in line with the user requirements collaboratively defined by HCPs, the informal caregivers, as well as the patients themselves during the project's first phase (which is coming to its end). Their daily activities in terms of motor function will be monitored by wearables, while both they and their caregivers will be enabled to provide input about their fluctuating condition; input from caregivers will be especially important in cases in which the patients themselves do not have a complete realisation of their condition, for example, during their cognitive fluctuations, or when they manifest dyskinesias, of which they may not be aware.

As observed in the previous sections, with regard to the brain diseases under study, SDM is largely defined with respect to decisions concerning medical treatments. However, the ALAMEDA pilots are not set up as interventional studies, meaning that treatment of participants in the pilots occurs in accordance with existing medical practices for PMSS patients. Instead, the ALAMEDA pilots are defined as observational studies in which the medical act of monitoring the evolution of the disease/recovery process is extended using technical means including wearable devices and software applications (a process generically called the 'Patient Data Collection Journey'). Thus, the general objective of the ALAMEDA SDM is to inform the patients about the available customisation points of the ALAMEDA monitoring process and to arrive at a decision on how their data collection journey and data interaction methods will look like within the ALAMEDA pilots. It is therefore a customisation and adaptation of the original SDM principals to the focus points of the ALAMEDA pilot studies, which are observational rather than interventional in nature.

During the first months of ALAMEDA, clinicians identified variables for continuous passive and discrete monitoring for the end users involved in the project. The selection of the clinical variables took into consideration several types of impairment and limitations linked to the PMSS. The variables cover motor, physical, emotional, cognitive and sleep conditions.

Use cases specification and selection was carried out with the aim to take into account all the features of the population expected to use the system. This is mandatory for the design of a system suitable for its users,

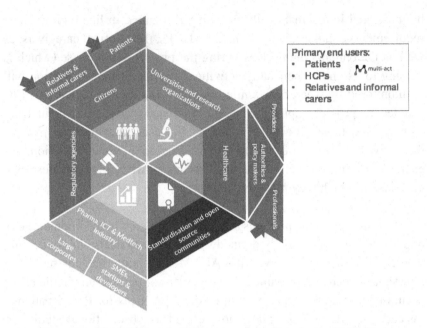

Figure 3.   ALAMEDA stakeholder categories with end users highlighted.

including requirements in terms of accessibility, usability and acquaintance to use technologies. The design of the overall system has been fully centred on users and their needs (Figure 3).

4.1. Patient engagement in ALAMEDA: Building on MULTI-ACT project legacy

As digital technology continues to evolve rapidly and healthcare providers and policymakers work hard to adapt, there is a high risk that the patient perspective may be lost. For this reason, ALAMEDA puts meaningful patient engagement at the top of its priorities and builds on the learnings of previous projects and experiences to ensure it is carried out in the most effective, participatory and purposeful way.

Specifically, ALAMEDA relies upon the participation of the Italian Multiple Sclerosis Society Foundation (FISM) as a key partner and former coordinator of the MULTI-ACT project.

MULTI-ACT is a three-year project funded within the H2020 Science with and for Society programme (May 2018–April 2021). The aim is to increase the impact of health research on people with brain disorders by providing a framework and tools for multi-stakeholder health research initiatives (such as EU-funded projects), allowing an effective cooperation of all the relevant stakeholders and the alignment of the results to the mission and agenda.

Over the last decade, patient engagement has become more important along with the democratisation of health sciences. Patients started to be engaged not only in a passive role, but also as co-researchers. In fact, they can share with other stakeholders their own experience of the disease, which translates into a form of knowledge that integrates with and enriches scientific knowledge (experiential knowledge).

MULTI-ACT has developed a strategic Collective Research Governance and Sustainability Model (which is freely available and accessible via a handy digital toolbox) in the area of brain diseases by using MS as the first case study. The project foresees patients as a key stakeholder in the health R&I process. Hence, the project aims to contribute to the development of the 'science with/of patient inputs' by providing guidelines for patient engagement in R&I (with) and by applying the patient-reported dimension in addition to the four research impact assessment dimensions (i.e. excellence, social impact, economic impact and adherence to the stated mission) of the MULTI-ACT model.

Specifically, with regard to patient engagement strategies and methodologies, MULTI-ACT has developed a set of guidelines which equip multi-stakeholder research initiatives with a tool to enable patient engagement actions into the R&I path at both programme and project levels.

The guidelines propose a roadmap to capture 'experiential knowledge' of patients (i.e. knowledge gained through lived experience that researchers may not have), to better understand how to draw on their experience and use the experience constructively for co-creation purposes. This way, MULTI-ACT aims at leveraging both patients and other stakeholders' experience and at raising their ability to co-create and participate in decision-making processes.

The MULTI-ACT guidelines indicate how to apply the project's patient engagement strategy within the activities of multi-stakeholder initiatives and are going to be used and contextualised in the frame of ALAMEDA.

As a first fundamental step, ALAMEDA has settled the Engagement Coordination Team (ECT) which, according to the guidelines, is aimed toward: '(i) creating commitment among the members and their community; (ii) moderating the dialogue between interdisciplinary and different (and sometimes competing) voices and experiences and settling a dispute resolution system; (iii) mitigating challenges such as ethical conflicts in protocol design, tokenism, power struggles, difficulties in recruiting different patients, additional time, cost; (iv) assuring that patients "feel valued" by facilitating team interaction and setting up an inclusive research environment' (MULTI-ACT Guidelines, 2020). This path is already being undertaken by relevant international multi-stakeholder health research initiatives whose promoters have embraced the MULTI-CT model such as the International Progressive MS Alliance.[2]

As for its composition, the ECT has been shaped in a way that ensures adequate representativeness to the three different disease-specific communities involved in ALAMEDA. Thus, it comprises one patient and one clinician from each of the three disease domains considered in the project, an ethics expert, a representative of the technological partners from Wellics Ltd and two representatives from FISM and WISE, respectively, in charge of coordination and implementing the patient engagement strategy and overseeing the whole process of stakeholder engagement along the project.

During its kick-off meeting, the participants have been provided with an in-depth introduction of the project's goals, ambitions and general stakeholder engagement principles as well as the explanation of the MULTI-ACT Patient Engagement Roadmap. The patient representatives were introduced to all research stages in which they could practically develop their contribution (design & plan, research execution, evaluation and translation to community) and were requested to reflect about their expectations towards the project's outcomes and the aspects of the research they felt they would more likely be able and comfortable to meaningfully contribute towards.

---

[2] https://www.progressivemsalliance.org/who-we-are/people-affected-by-ms-engagement-coordination-team/.

In order to operationalise the MULTI-ACT guidelines into the ALAMEDA context, a series of steps have been identified and agreed to with the aim of translating the indications prescribed by the guidelines into feasible actions within the ALAMEDA work plan (Table 1).

The second ECT meeting was indeed an important opportunity to share the outcomes of local engagement activities run so far at the level of pilot sites, discuss preliminary findings, and agree on the next steps.

At that time the three Local Community Groups had been constituted in Italy, Romania and Greece, respectively, including patients, caregivers and clinicians involved in the planning and delivery of care and rehabilitation services in the three neurological disease domains of MS, stroke and PD.

Among the topic discussed, the different consultation modalities and tools used in the three settings were described. While FISM (Italy) and SUUB (Romania) utilised individual interviews and focus groups as main methods, in Greece (NKUA) the team opted for using a remote and asynchronous feedback collection strategy (via email and online forms). Also, notable good practices have emerged, e.g. in the selection of patients belonging to the Italian LCG where specific attention has been paid to gender balance as well as representativeness in terms of diversified personal profiles with different educational and professional background and family responsibilities.

The first iterations of the LCG engagement have been basically meant to gather the direct insights from their members on the questions to be asked via questionnaires with a view to focus stronger attention on symptoms and circumstances which, according to the experiential knowledge of patients with their conditions, may represent warning signs of potential worsening or relapse 'red flags'. In addition, preferences in relation to the user-interface interaction modalities, length and frequency of measurements, or the willingness to allow the capture of face image during the interactions so as to make emotional sensing and analytics possible, have been collected.

So far, the work done to involve patients has been much appreciated. Importantly, all patients have shown trust towards the team they are working along with. The patients/caregivers are reportedly willing to provide feedback and being involved in research, though still some doubt arose

Table 1. Operationalisation of the MULTI-ACT patient engagement guidelines within ALAMEDA.

Step of the R&I path	Patient engagement activities suggested by the MULTI-ACT guidelines	ALAMEDA translation into action
Design & plan	• Patients are engaged to suggest objectives, endpoints and outcomes of research. • Patients are engaged to define the relevance and acceptability of proposed research to patient community.	• ECT local representatives act as bridges between project and local realities. • ECT members are trained to reach out to the relevant community. • ECT and LCG members provide inputs on the prioritisation of research items and evaluation plans.
Research	• Patients are engaged in the *development and monitoring of research at Project Level* (e.g. collaborating for ICT device development, for the enrolment to increase participation and decrease drop-down, to increase compliance with protocols and facilitate data collection...).	• ECT and LCG members may be the first testers of ALAMEDA devices and softwares. • ECT members facilitate communications between patients and technical partners.
Evaluation	• Patients are engaged in discussing about *new methods to measure the impact of research and align results* to the mission/agenda. • Patients are engaged in *the assessment of new approaches* and products arising from research. • Patients are engaged in research and impact assessment reports.	• Patients and caregivers are invited to evaluate the devices employed in ALAMEDA (usability, accessibility, safety, etc.), the timing of use, their perspectives about simultaneous use of 1+ devices.
Translation to community	• Patients are engaged in *shaping the 'translation strategy' of research results* to easy-to-use and easy-to-understand (lay) material and in communication activities to disseminate the research results. • Patients are engaged in advocacy to leverage uptake of research results.	• The ECT and LCG members are mobilised to support the communication and dissemination efforts via their local or national associations.

regarding their perception of the added value of their contribution which in some cases makes patients hesitant about the necessity of their engagement.

In this regard, several ECT participants agreed that it may be too early to perceive a real return of engagement as the project is not mature enough to report tangible results to the LCG members. However, as a follow-up action, the participants agree that it will be crucial to keep the LCG members constantly informed about progress and make them aware of how their inputs are concretely helping shape the system. Also, giving them the chance to access the prototypes and demos and test the devices, although they won't be among the patients recruited to take part in the study formally, will be core to increasing their comprehension and sense of utility.

Both in FISM and NKUA experience, the intermediation of the respective patient association has proven very valuable so far, both in ALAMEDA and other projects. SUUB is for the moment not connected to any association at the local level, however, the team is investigating the chance to connect with the national Romanian association.

In general, the importance of adapting the engagement approach to the local context is clearly emerging, using existing channels and networks that already effectively work for patients and with which they feel comfortable to informally share their lived experiences, such as in Facebook groups, Whatsapp chats and others.

5. Future Delivery

The activities conducted in the first year and a half of the ALAMEDA project have built a solid innovative approach to participatory design and implementation of digital health solutions for brain health assessment, thus setting the scene for the research experiments and evaluation to be conducted during the second and third project's years. After having identified the disease-specific use cases, designed the relevant *personas* — as a prerequisite to determine the inclusion criteria for patient recruitment and onboarding in the ALAMEDA study — and defined the technical and functional requirements, the team has then focused on grasping a better understanding of the broader healthcare scenarios where the ALAMEDA system is going to be tested, and highlighted specific local features, main differences and similarities. To this end, this chapter provides an in-depth overview of the key aspects of each disease-specific care journey, which in turn represent important grounds for reflection for the future deployment and scaling up plans.

The first part of the document highlights relevant commonalities between the use cases identified for PD and MS due to the chronicity and progression of the conditions over time which characterise both. The current absence of a cure, the need to cope with very diversified and broad range of symptoms as well as the adverse effects induced by pharmacological treatments, are elements of high concern for the patients and their carers. All of the above make the two disease domains extremely relevant for the potential progress in enhanced and increasingly personalised care and rehabilitation that real-life health monitoring and predictive tools can bring. On the other hand, stroke patients suffer from an acute episode which might pose very diverse consequences to their health and well-being depending on the gravity of the attack and the timeliness of the intervention. The recovery towards full or partial autonomy and functionality in tandem with the risk of suffering another episode is then strictly dependent upon a complex set of factors, including the effectiveness of the rehabilitation programme and the secondary prevention measures recommended by the clinicians and undertaken by the patients, such as lifestyle changes and health-promoting behaviours. Therefore, even in the stroke case, the continuous monitoring of patients leading to accumulation of large number of objective measurements ('big data') can provide a complementary and precious source of information that can span across large periods of time of monitoring in real-life conditions of the patients thus allowing to assess and eventually review rehabilitation and secondary prevention plans. Monitoring and reporting back to the patients, even after the rehabilitation goals are reached, would help and provide guidance to the 'former' patients and their caregivers (self-reporting, self-monitoring) to keep track of their well-being, lifestyle, diet, and activity changes they accomplished during their rehabilitation period. Thus, apart from building a time-dependent personalised record, which will be continuously built up with a view to minimise invasiveness so as to promote the usability by the patients, and which will also be available to the carers and medical personnel, they will be able to gain insight about any deviation, across time, of any relevant aspect of their quality of life. Either disease-specific or non-disease-specific indicators will be monitored and will alert patients to prompt early adaptation or even reach out for help (either to their medical doctor or their carers — who would also be aware of the situation).

The complexity of the care system and multiplicity of specialities and professionals involved in the healthcare of patients, and provision of support to their caregivers, is transversal to the three diseases. Though the degree of actual integration and the ease of navigation across different providers and services vary considerably across countries and local settings. Similarly, the involvement of patients in decision-making, as well as their engagement in research and healthcare services' redesign and enhancement, has been progressing with different speed and intensity.

From the consultation with local clinicians leading the ALAMEDA pilots, important differences emerge also in terms of the typology and role of the providers and professionals involved across the healthcare continuum.

The Greek pilot is settled in the Special Outpatient Clinic of Parkinson's Disease and Related Movement Disorders of the neurology department of a reference public hospital of the capital Athens which covers several specialities. The patients with PD are usually most in need of specialised neurologists and nurses, psychologists, neuropsychologists, nutritionists, SW and psychiatrists. In this sense, the Clinic shows quite a high degree of interdisciplinarity, though the patients are still often referred to external healthcare providers when they need specific assistance from other specialists.

In the Italian validation scenario, instead, the central actor involved in the pilot is a rehabilitation clinic for PwMS, thus representing one of the core 'allied' healthcare entities participating in the broad ecosystem of MS healthcare service providers. In this case, the added value brought by ALAMEDA will not directly impact the healthcare services provided by the public providers (e.g. the hospital neurologists in charge of the medical assessment and pharmacological treatment plan). Though demonstrating its usefulness and effectiveness could open new routes for strengthened cooperation and integration. Ultimately, the large amount of data collected and the valuable information retrieved from the continuous health monitoring of the patients may not only be relevant to help the clinic rehabilitation specialists finetune the personalised rehabilitation plan of each patient but also provide precious information that coupled with imaging and other data sources could provide the neurologists in charge with a better understanding of disease progression and treatment effects.

Last, in the Romanian pilot settings, patients are being recruited by the emergency department of a reference hospital of the capital Bucharest where they are treated in the acute stroke phase and receive in-patient rehabilitation assistance. The ALAMEDA system will then be particularly useful for the clinicians to perform closer and continuous monitoring of the patients after discharge and obtain information about the evolution of their health conditions and their recovery. However, further opportunities for deployment and scaling up are envisaged in the potential engagement and coordination with outpatient clinics and other service providers, external to the hospital, to which the patients are referred when discharged to continue their rehabilitation program.

In conclusion, in all the three disease domains, an emerging specific area which demands further research and development is indeed patient remote monitoring, which is at the core of ALAMEDA, a result which is consistent across literature and has been recently highlighted by European institutions as one of the breakthrough health innovation strands (European Innovation Council (EIC) & European Innovation Council and SMEs Executive Agency (EISMEA), 2022) in the continuous attempt to optimise the healthcare continuum. Furthermore, the preliminary positive outcomes from the end user engagement strategy call for further and larger experiments in this direction and highlight that patients' stronger and earlier involvement in the innovation process is the keystone to securing higher acceptance, usability as well as promoting a paradigmatic shift towards proactive civic participation in R&I. In this direction, ALAMEDA envisions that the persons affected by the diseases will not only be advisors in the R&I process, but they can also act as ambassadors that engage corresponding communities in order to mobilise and capture experiential knowledge of larger groups of people living with the same conditions.

References

Adeoye, O., Nyström, K. V., Yavagal, D. R., Luciano, J., Nogueira, R. G., Zorowitz, R. D., Khalessi, A. A., Bushnell, C., Barsan, W. G., Panagos, P., Alberts, M. J., Tiner, A. C., Schwamm, L. H. & Jauch, E. C. (2019) Recommendations for the establishment of stroke systems of care: A 2019 update. *Stroke*, 50(7), e187–e210. Available at: https://doi.org/10.1161/STR.0000000000000173.

Aguilar, M. I. (2015) Acute ischemic stroke and transient ischemic attack. In: Demaerschalk, B. M. & Wingerchuk, D. M. (eds.) *Evidence-Based Neurology: Management of Neurological Disorders*. Available at: https://doi.org/10.1002/9781119067344.ch6.

Albanese, A., Di Fonzo, A., Fetoni, V., Franzini, A., Gennuso, M., Molini, G., Pacchetti, C., Priori, A., Riboldazzi, G., Volonté, M. A. & Calandrella, D. (2020) Design and operation of the Lombardy Parkinson's Disease Network. *Frontiers in Neurology*, 11, 573. Available at: https://doi.org/10.3389/fneur.2020.00573.

Armstrong, M. J. (2017) Shared decision-making in stroke: An evolving approach to improved patient care. *Stroke and Vascular Neurology*, 2(2), 84–87. Available at: https://doi.org/10.1136/svn-2017-000081.

Armstrong, M. J., Shulman, L. M., Vandigo, J. & Mullins, C. D. (2016) Patient engagement and shared decision-making: What do they look like in neurology practice? *Neurology Clinical Practice*, 6(2), 190–197. Available at: https://doi.org/10.1212/CPJ.0000000000000240.

Ben-Zacharia, A., Adamson, M., Boyd, A., Hardeman, P., Smrtka, J., Walker, B. & Walker, T. (2018) Impact of shared decision making on disease-modifying drug adherence in multiple sclerosis. *International Journal of MS Care*, 20(6), 287–297. Available at: https://doi.org/10.7224/1537-2073.2017-070.

Bientzle, M., Kimmerle, J., Eggeling, M., Cebi, I., Weiss, D. & Gharabaghi, A. (2020) Evidence-based decision aid for patients with Parkinson disease: Protocol for interview study, online survey, and two randomized controlled trials. *JMIR Research Protocols*, 9(7), e17482. Available at: https://doi.org/10.2196/17482.

Bird, M., McGillion, M., Chambers, E. M., *et al.* (2021) A generative co-design framework for healthcare innovation: Development and application of an end-user engagement framework. *Research Involvement and Engagement*, 7, 12. Available at: https://doi.org/10.1186/s40900-021-00252-7.

Bisson, E. J., Finlayson, M. L., Ekuma, O., Marrie, R. A. & Leslie, W. D. (2019) Accuracy of FRAX® in people with multiple sclerosis. *Journal of Bone and Mineral Research*, 34(6), 1095–1100. Available at: https://doi.org/10.1002/jbmr.3682.

Bloem, B. R. & Munneke, M. (2014) Revolutionising management of chronic disease: The ParkinsonNet approach. *BMJ* (Clinical research ed.), 348, g1838. Available at: https://doi.org/10.1136/bmj.g1838.

Bloem, B. R., Henderson, E. J., Dorsey, E. R., Okun, M. S., Okubadejo, N., Chan, P., Andrejack, J., Darweesh, S. & Munneke, M. (2020) Integrated and patient-centred management of Parkinson's disease: A network model for reshaping chronic neurological care. *The Lancet. Neurology*, 19(7), 623–634. Available at: https://doi.org/10.1016/S1474-4422(20)30064-8.

Bloem, B. R., Henderson, E. J., Dorsey, E. R., Okun, M. S., Okubadejo, N., Chan, P., Andrejack, J., Darweesh, S. & Munneke, M. (2020) Patient-centred management of Parkinson's disease — Authors' reply. *The Lancet. Neurology*, 19(11), 889–890. Available at: https://doi.org/10.1016/S1474-4422(20)30360-4.

Bloem, B. R., Okun, M. S. & Klein, C. (2021) Parkinson's disease. *Lancet (London, England)*, 397(10291), 2284–2303. Available at: https://doi.org/10.1016/S0140-6736(21)00218-X.

Bodenheimer, T. & Sinsky, C. (2014) From triple to quadruple aim: Care of the patient requires care of the provider. *Annals of Family Medicine*, 12(6), 573–576. Available at: https://doi.org/10.1370/afm.1713.

Bonkhoff, A. K. & Grefkes, C. (2021) Precision medicine in stroke: Towards personalized outcome predictions using artificial intelligence. *Brain: A Journal of Neurology*, awab439. Advance online publication. Available at: https://doi.org/10.1093/brain/awab439.

Brichetto, G. & Zaratin, P. (2020) Measuring outcomes that matter most to people with multiple sclerosis: The role of patient-reported outcomes. *Current Opinion in Neurology*, 33(3), 295–299. Available at: https://doi.org/10.1097/WCO.0000000000000821.

Brichetto, G., Monti Bragadin, M., Fiorini, S., Battaglia, M. A., Konrad, G., Ponzio, M., Pedullà, L., Verri, A., Barla, A. & Tacchino, A. (2020) The hidden information in patient-reported outcomes and clinician-assessed outcomes: Multiple sclerosis as a proof of concept of a machine learning approach. *Neurological Sciences*, 41(2), 459–462. Available at: https://doi.org/10.1007/s10072-019-04093-x.

Brichetto, G., Pedullà, L., Podda, J. & Tacchino, A. (2019) Beyond center-based testing: Understanding and improving functioning with wearable technology in MS. *Multiple Sclerosis (Houndmills, Basingstoke, England)*, 25(10), 1402–1411. Available at: https://doi.org/10.1177/1352458519857075.

British Society of Rehabilitation Medicine (2003) Rehabilitation following acquired brain injury: National clinical guidelines. Physicians RCo.

Brown, H., Gabriele, S. & White, J. (2018) Physician and patient treatment decision-making in relapsing-remitting multiple sclerosis in Europe and the USA. *Neurodegenerative Disease Management*, 8(6), 371–376. Available at: https://doi.org/10.2217/nmt-2018-0023.

Chitnis, T. & Prat, A. (2020) A roadmap to precision medicine for multiple sclerosis. *Multiple Sclerosis Journal*, 26(5), 522–532. Available at: https://doi.org/10.1177/1352458519881558.

Clarke, D. J. & Forster, A. (2015) Improving post-stroke recovery: The role of the multidisciplinary health care team. *Journal of Multidisciplinary Healthcare*, 8, 433–442. Available at: https://doi.org/10.2147/JMDH.S68764.

Colligan, E., Metzler, A. & Tiryaki, E. (2017) Shared decision-making in multiple sclerosis. *Multiple Sclerosis (Houndmills, Basingstoke, England)*, 23(2), 185–190. Available at: https://doi.org/10.1177/1352458516671204.

De Panfilis, L., Veronese, S., Bruzzone, M., Cascioli, M., Gajofatto, A., Grasso, M. G., Kruger, P., Lugaresi, A., Manson, L., Montepietra, S., Patti, F., Pucci, E., Solaro, C., Giordano, A. & Solari, A. (2021) Study protocol on advance care planning in multiple sclerosis (ConCure-SM): Intervention construction and multicentre feasibility trial. *BMJ Open*, 11(8), e052012. Available at: https://doi.org/10.1136/bmjopen-2021-052012.

Desborough, J., Brunoro, C., Parkinson, A., Chisholm, K., Elisha, M., Drew, J., Fanning, V., Lueck, C., Bruestle, A., Cook, M., Suominen, H., Tricoli, A., Henschke, A. & Phillips, C. (2020) 'It struck at the heart of who I thought I was': A meta-synthesis of the qualitative literature examining the experiences of people with multiple sclerosis. *Health Expectations*, 23(5), 1007–1027. Available at: https://doi.org/10.1111/hex.13093.

Di Luca, M., *et al.* (2020) Rethinking MS in Europe: Prioritising timely, integrated care for people with multiple sclerosis. *Journal of Clinical Neurology and Neurosurgery*, 3(2020), 119. Available at: https://doi.org/10.37421/jcnn.2020.3.119.

Dillenseger, A., Weidemann, M. L., Trentzsch, K., Inojosa, H., Haase, R., Schriefer, D., Voigt, I., Scholz, M., Akgün, K. & Ziemssen, T. (2021) Digital biomarkers in multiple sclerosis. *Brain Sciences*, 11(11), 1519. Available at: https://doi.org/10.3390/brainsci11111519.

Dorsey, E. R., Sherer, T., Okun, M. S. & Bloem, B. R. (2020) *Ending Parkinson's Disease: A Prescription for Action*. Public Affairs, New York, NY.

Dorsey, E. R., Constantinescu, R., Thompson, J. P., Biglan, K. M., Holloway, R. G., Kieburtz, K., Marshall, F. J., Ravina, B. M., Schifitto, G., Siderowf, A. & Tanner, C. M. (2007) Projected number of people with Parkinson disease in the most populous nations, 2005 through 2030. *Neurology*, 68(5), 384–386. Available at: https://doi.org/10.1212/01.wnl.0000247740.47667.03.

Dorsey, E. R., Sherer, T., Okun, M. S. & Bloem, B. R. (2018) The emerging evidence of the Parkinson pandemic. *Journal of Parkinson's Disease*, 8(S1), S3–S8. Available at: https://doi.org/10.3233/JPD-181474.

Dorsey, E. R., Voss, T. S., Shprecher, D. R., Deuel, L. M., Beck, C. A., Gardiner, I. F., Coles, M. A., Burns, R. S., Marshall, F. J. & Biglan, K. M. (2010) A U.S. survey of patients with Parkinson's disease: Satisfaction with medical care and support groups. *Movement Disorders*, 25(13), 2128–2135. Available at: https://doi.org/10.1002/mds.23160.

Duddy, M., Lee, M., Pearson, O., Nikfekr, E., Chaudhuri, A., Percival, F., Roberts, M. & Whitlock, C. (2014) The UK patient experience of relapse in multiple sclerosis treated with first disease modifying therapies. *Multiple Sclerosis and Related Disorders*, 3(4), 450–456. Available at: https://doi.org/10.1016/j.msard.2014.02.006.

EFNA (2021) Addressing the impact of COVID-19 on the lives of people living with neurological disorders. Available at: https://www.efna.net/wp-content/uploads/2021/06/EFNA-Report_Final-.pdf.

Eggers, C., Dano, R., Schill, J., Fink, G. R., Hellmich, M., Timmermann, L. & CPN Study Group (2018) Patient-centered integrated healthcare improves quality of life in Parkinson's disease patients: A randomized controlled trial. *Journal of Neurology*, 265(4), 764–773. Available at: https://doi.org/10.1007/s00415-018-8761-7.

Elwyn, G., Frosch, D., Thomson, R., Joseph-Williams, N., Lloyd, A., Kinnersley, P., Cording, E., Tomson, D., Dodd, C., Rollnick, S., Edwards, A. & Barry, M. (2012) Shared decision making: A model for clinical practice. *Journal of General Internal Medicine*, 27(10), 1361–1367. Available at: https://doi.org/10.1007/s11606-012-2077-6.

Eskyte, I., Manzano, A., Pepper, G., Pavitt, S., Ford, H., Bekker, H., Chataway, J., Schmierer, K., Meads, D., Webb, E. & Potrata, B. (2019) Understanding treatment decisions from the perspective of people with relapsing remitting multiple sclerosis: A critical interpretive synthesis. *Multiple Sclerosis and Related Disorders*, 27, 370–377. Available at: https://doi.org/10.1016/j.msard.2018.11.016.

Espay, A. J., Bonato, P., Nahab, F. B., Maetzler, W., Dean, J. M., Klucken, J., Eskofier, B. M., Merola, A., Horak, F., Lang, A. E., Reilmann, R., Giuffrida, J., Nieuwboer, A., Horne, M., Little, M. A., Litvan, I., Simuni, T., Dorsey, E. R., Burack, M. A., Kubota, K., … & Movement Disorders Society Task Force on Technology (2016) Technology in Parkinson's disease: Challenges and opportunities. *Movement Disorders*, 31(9), 1272–1282. Available at: https://doi.org/10.1002/mds.26642.

European Commission (2021) Health Technology Assessment: Commission welcomes the adoption of new rules to improve access to innovative technologies, Press release, 13 December 2021, Brussels. Available at: https://ec.europa.eu/commission/presscorner/detail/en/IP_21_6771.

European Innovation Council and SMEs Executive Agency, Lopatka, M., Pólvora, A., Manimaaran, S., *et al.* (2022) Identification of emerging technologies and breakthrough innovations. Publications Office of the European Union. Available at: https://data.europa.eu/doi/10.2826/06288.

Ferguson, C. & Hendriks, J. (2017) Partnering with patients in shared decision-making for stroke prevention in atrial fibrillation. *European Journal of Cardiovascular Nursing*, 16(3), 178–180. Available at: https://doi.org/10.1177/1474515116685193.

Ferreira, J. J., Katzenschlager, R., Bloem, B. R., Bonuccelli, U., Burn, D., Deuschl, G., Dietrichs, E., Fabbrini, G., Friedman, A., Kanovsky, P., Kostic, V., Nieuwboer, A., Odin, P., Poewe, W., Rascol, O., Sampaio, C., Schüpbach, M., Tolosa, E., Trenkwalder, C., Schapira, A., Berardelli, A. and Oertel, W. H. (2013) Summary of the recommendations of the EFNS/MDS-ES review on therapeutic management of Parkinson's disease. *European Journal of Neurology*, 20, 5–15. Available at: https://doi.org/10.1111/j.1468-1331.2012.03866.x.

GBD 2016 Neurology Collaborators (2019) Global, regional, and national burden of neurological disorders, 1990-2016: A systematic analysis for the Global Burden of Disease Study 2016. *The Lancet. Neurology*, 18(5), 459–480. Available at: https://doi.org/10.1016/S1474-4422(18)30499-X.

Gorelick, P. B. (2019) The global burden of stroke: Persistent and disabling. *The Lancet. Neurology*, 18(5), 417–418. Available at: https://doi.org/10.1016/S1474-4422(19)30030-4.

Grau-Pellicer, M., Lalanza, J. F., Jovell-Fernández, E. & Capdevila, L. (2020) Impact of mHealth technology on adherence to healthy PA after stroke: A randomized study. *Topics in Stroke Rehabilitation*, 27(5), 354–368. Available at: https://doi.org/10.1080/10749357.2019.1691816.

Gustavsson, A., Svensson, M., Jacobi, F., Allgulander, C., Alonso, J., Beghi, E., Dodel, R., Ekman, M., Faravelli, C., Fratiglioni, L., Gannon, B., Jones, D. H., Jennum, P., Jordanova, A., Jönsson, L., Karampampa, K., Knapp, M., Kobelt, G., Kurth, T., Lieb, R., … CDBE2010 Study Group (2011) Cost of disorders of the brain in Europe 2010. *European Neuropsychopharmacology*, 21(10), 718–779. Available at: https://doi.org/10.1016/j.euroneuro.2011.08.008.

Hancock, N. J., Collins, K., Dorer, C., Wolf, S. L., Bayley, M. & Pomeroy, V. M. (2019) Evidence-based practice 'on-the-go': Using ViaTherapy as a tool to enhance clinical decision making in upper limb rehabilitation after stroke, a quality improvement initiative. *BMJ Open Quality*, 8(3), e000592. Available at: https://doi.org/10.1136/bmjoq-2018-000592.

Harris, N. R. & Sthapit, D. (2016) Towards a personalised rehabilitation system for post stroke treatment. In: *2016 IEEE Sensors Applications Symposium (SAS).* IEEE Press, pp. 1–5. Available at: https://doi.org/10.1109/SAS.2016.7479848.

Henschke, A., Desborough, J., Parkinson, A., Brunoro, C., Fanning, V., Lueck, C., Brew-Sam, N., Brüstle, A., Drew, J., Chisholm, K., Elisha, M., Suominen, H., Tricoli, A., Phillips, C. & Cook, M. (2021) Personalizing medicine and technologies to address the experiences and needs of people with multiple sclerosis. *Journal of Personalized Medicine*, 11(8), 791. Available at: https://doi.org/10.3390/jpm11080791.

Herrgårdh, T., Madai, V. I., Kelleher, J. D., Magnusson, R., Gustafsson, M., Milani, L., Gennemark, P. & Cedersund, G. (2021) Hybrid modelling for stroke care: Review and suggestions of new approaches for risk assessment and simulation of scenarios. *NeuroImage. Clinical*, 31, 102694. Available at: https://doi.org/10.1016/j.nicl.2021.102694.

Hinman, J. D., Rost, N. S., Leung, T. W., Montaner, J., Muir, K. W., Brown, S., Arenillas, J. F., Feldmann, E. & Liebeskind, D. S. (2017) Principles of precision medicine in stroke. *Journal of Neurology, Neurosurgery, and Psychiatry*, 88(1), 54–61. Available at: https://doi.org/10.1136/jnnp-2016-314587.

Hvid, L. G., Gaemelke, T., Dalgas, U., Slipsager, M. K., Rasmussen, P. V., Petersen, T., Nørgaard, M., Skjerbaek, A. G. & Boesen, F. (2021) Personalised inpatient multidisciplinary rehabilitation elicits clinically relevant improvements in physical function in patients with multiple sclerosis — The Danish MS Hospitals Rehabilitation Study. *Multiple Sclerosis Journal — Experimental, Translational and Clinical.* Available at: https://doi.org/10.1177/2055217321989384.

Iodice, F., Romoli, M., Giometto, B., Clerico, M., Tedeschi, G., Bonavita, S., Leocani, L., Lavorgna, L. & Digital Technologies, Web and Social Media Study Group of the Italian Society of Neurology (2021) Stroke and digital technology: A wake-up call from COVID-19 pandemic. *Neurological Sciences*, 42(3), 805–809. Available at: https://doi.org/10.1007/s10072-020-04993-3.

Jauch, E. C., Saver, J. L., Adams, H. P., Jr, Bruno, A., Connors, J. J., Demaerschalk, B. M., Khatri, P., McMullan, P. W., Jr, Qureshi, A. I., Rosenfield, K., Scott, P. A., Summers, D. R., Wang, D. Z., Wintermark, M.,

Yonas, H., American Heart Association Stroke Council, Council on Cardiovascular Nursing, Council on Peripheral Vascular Disease, & Council on Clinical Cardiology (2013) Guidelines for the early management of patients with acute ischemic stroke: A guideline for healthcare professionals from the American Heart Association/American Stroke Association. *Stroke*, 44(3), 870–947. Available at: https://doi.org/10.1161/STR.0b013e318284056a.

Kanavos, P., Tinelli, M., Efthymiadou, O., Visintin, E., Grimaccia, F. & Mossman, J. (2016) Towards better outcomes in multiple sclerosis by addressing policy change: The International MultiPlE Sclerosis Study (IMPrESS). Available at: https://www.lse.ac.uk/business/consulting/reports/towards-better-outcomes-in-ms.

Kanzler, C. M., Lamers, I., Feys, P., *et al.* (2022) Personalized prediction of rehabilitation outcomes in multiple sclerosis: A proof-of-concept using clinical data, digital health metrics, and machine learning. *Medical & Biological Engineering & Computing*, 60, 249–261. Available at: https://doi.org/10.1007/s11517-021-02467-y.

Kes, V. B., Cengić, L., Cesarik, M., Tomas, A. J., Zavoreo, I., Matovina, L. Z., Corić, L., Drnasin, S. & Demarin, V. (2013) Quality of life in patients with multiple sclerosis. *Acta Clinica Croatica*, 52(1), 107–111.

Kim, G. J., Kim, H., Fletcher, J., Voelbel, G. T., Goverover, Y., Chen, P., O'Dell, M. W. & Genova, H. M. (2021) The differential impact of the COVID-19 pandemic on healthcare utilization disruption for community-dwelling individuals with and without acquired brain injury. *Archives of Rehabilitation Research and Clinical Translation*, 100176. Advance online publication. Available at: https://doi.org/10.1016/j.arrct.2021.100176.

Kim, J., Thrift, A. G., Nelson, M. R., Bladin, C. F. & Cadilhac, D. A. (2015) Personalized medicine and stroke prevention: Where are we? *Vascular Health and Risk Management*, 11, 601–611. Available at: https://doi.org/10.2147/VHRM.S77571.

Klop, G. & Rutte, A. (2021) *Value-Based Healthcare: The Answer to Our Future Healthcare Challenges?* Available at: https://www.europeanallianceforvalue-inhealth.eu/wp-content/uploads/2021/06/Value-Based-Healthcare-The-answer-to-our-future-healthcare-challenges_a_Vintura_report.pdf.

Klucken, J., Krüger, R., Schmidt, P. & Bloem, B. R. (2018) Management of Parkinson's disease 20 years from now: Towards digital health pathways. *Journal of Parkinson's Disease*, 8(S1), S85–S94. Available at: https://doi.org/10.3233/JPD-181519.

Kobelt, G., Thompson, A., Berg, J., Gannedahl, M., Eriksson, J., MSCOI Study Group, & European Multiple Sclerosis Platform (2017) New insights into the burden and costs of multiple sclerosis in Europe. *Multiple Sclerosis (Houndmills, Basingstoke, England)*, 23(8), 1123–1136. Available at: https://doi.org/10.1177/1352458517694432.

Lublin, F. D. & Reingold, S. C. (1996) Defining the clinical course of multiple sclerosis: Results of an international survey. National Multiple Sclerosis Society (USA) Advisory Committee on Clinical Trials of New Agents in Multiple Sclerosis. *Neurology*, 46(4), 907–911.

Luengo-Fernandez, R., Violato, M., Candio, P. & Leal, J. (2020) Economic burden of stroke across Europe: A population-based cost analysis. *European Stroke Journal*, 5(1), 17–25. Available at: https://doi.org/10.1177/2396987319883160.

Luis-Martínez, R., Monje, M., Antonini, A., Sánchez-Ferro, Á. & Mestre, T. A. (2020) Technology-enabled care: Integrating multidisciplinary care in Parkinson's disease through digital technology. *Frontiers in Neurology*, 11, 575975. Available at: https://doi.org/10.3389/fneur.2020.575975.

Manacorda, T., Bandiera, P., Terzuoli, F., Ponzio, M., Brichetto, G., Zaratin, P., Bezzini, D. & Battaglia, M. A. (2021) Impact of the COVID-19 pandemic on persons with multiple sclerosis: Early findings from a survey on disruptions in care and self-reported outcomes. *Journal of Health Services Research & Policy*, 26(3), 189–197. Available at: https://doi.org/10.1177/1355819620975069.

Marrie, R. A. (2017) Comorbidity in multiple sclerosis: Implications for patient care. *Nature Reviews. Neurology*, 13(6), 375–382. Available at: https://doi.org/10.1038/nrneurol.2017.33.

Massachusetts eHealth Institute (2017) Caregivers and digital health: A survey of trends and attitudes of Massachusetts family caregivers, June 2017. Available at: https://mehi.masstech.org/2017-caregivers-and-digital-health-report.

Montalban, X., Gold, R., Thompson, A. J., Otero-Romero, S., Amato, M. P., Chandraratna, D., Clanet, M., Comi, G., Derfuss, T., Fazekas, F., Hartung, H. P., Havrdova, E., Hemmer, B., Kappos, L., Liblau, R., Lubetzki, C., Marcus, E., Miller, D. H., Olsson, T., Pilling, S., … & Zipp, F. (2018) ECTRIMS/EAN Guideline on the pharmacological treatment of people with multiple sclerosis. *Multiple Sclerosis (Houndmills, Basingstoke, England)*, 24(2), 96–120. Available at: https://doi.org/10.1177/1352458517751049.

Moral Torres, E., Fernández Fernández, Ó., Carrascal Rueda, P., Ruiz-Beato, E., Estella Pérez, E., Manzanares Estrada, R., Gómez-García, T., Jiménez, M., Hidalgo-Vega, Á. & Merino, M. (2020) Social value of a set of proposals for the ideal approach of multiple sclerosis within the Spanish National Health System: A social return on investment study. *BMC Health Services Research*, 20(1), 84. Available at: https://doi.org/10.1186/s12913-020-4946-8.

Mowry, E. M., Bermel, R. A., Williams, J. R., Benzinger, T., de Moor, C., Fisher, E., Hersh, C. M., Hyland, M. H., Izbudak, I., Jones, S. E., Kieseier, B. C., Kitzler, H. H., Krupp, L., Lui, Y. W., Montalban, X., Naismith, R. T., Nicholas, J. A., Pellegrini, F., Rovira, A., Schulze, M., ... & Rudick, R. A. (2020) Harnessing real-world data to inform decision-making: Multiple sclerosis partners advancing technology and health solutions (MS PATHS). *Frontiers in Neurology*, 11, 632. Available at: https://doi.org/10.3389/fneur.2020.00632.

Muangpaisan, W., Mathews, A., Hori, H. & Seidel, D. (2011) A systematic review of the worldwide prevalence and incidence of Parkinson's disease. *Journal of the Medical Association of Thailand = Chotmaihet thangphaet*, 94(6), 749–755.

MULTI-ACT (2020) Guidelines for Patient Engagement in Health Research & Innovation, Short publishable version, 2020, May 30. Available at: https://www.multiact.eu/wp-content/uploads/2020/06/MULTI-ACT-Patient-Engagement-Guidelines-Short-v0.1_compressed.pdf.

Murray, C. J., Vos, T., Lozano, R., Naghavi, M., Flaxman, A. D., Michaud, C., Ezzati, M., Shibuya, K., Salomon, J. A., Abdalla, S., Aboyans, V., Abraham, J., Ackerman, I., Aggarwal, R., Ahn, S. Y., Ali, M. K., Alvarado, M., Anderson, H. R., Anderson, L. M., Andrews, K. G., ... & Memish, Z. A. (2012) Disability-adjusted life years (DALYs) for 291 diseases and injuries in 21 regions, 1990-2010: A systematic analysis for the Global Burden of Disease Study 2010. *Lancet (London, England)*, 380(9859), 2197–2223. Available at: https://doi.org/10.1016/S0140-6736(12)61689-4.

Nardini, C., Osmani, V., Cormio, P. G., Frosini, A., Turrini, M., Lionis, C., Neumuth, T., Ballensiefen, W., Borgonovi, E. & D'Errico, G. (2021) The evolution of personalized healthcare and the pivotal role of European regions in its implementation. *Personalized Medicine*, 18(3), 283–294. Available at: https://doi.org/10.2217/pme-2020-0115.

National Institute for Health and Care Excellence (2017) Parkinson's disease in adults. (Nice guideline NG71). Available at: https://www.nice.org.uk/guidance/ng71.

NHS (2018) RightCare scenario: The variation between sub-optimal and optimal pathways. Sarah's story: Parkinson's. Available at: https://www.england.nhs.uk/rightcare/wp-content/uploads/sites/40/2018/02/sarahs-story-parkinsons-full-narrative.pdf.

Nijhuis, F., Elwyn, G., Bloem, B. R., Post, B. & Faber, M. J. (2018) Improving shared decision-making in advanced Parkinson's disease: Protocol of a mixed methods feasibility study. *Pilot and Feasibility Studies*, 4, 94. https://doi.org/10.1186/s40814-018-0286-4.

OECD (2019) Measuring what matters: The Patient Reported Indicator Surveys, 2019 Status Report. Available at: https://www.oecd.org/health/health-systems/Measuring-what-matters-the-Patient-Reported-Indicator-Surveys.pdf.

O'Neill, D., Horgan, F., Hickey, A. & McGee, H. (2008) Long term outcome of stroke: Stroke is a chronic disease with acute events. *BMJ* (Clinical research ed.), 336(7642), 461. Available at: https://doi.org/10.1136/bmj.39500.434086.1F.

Ovadia-Caro, S., Khalil, A. A., Sehm, B., Villringer, A., Nikulin, V. V. & Nazarova, M. (2019) Predicting the response to non-invasive brain stimulation in stroke. *Frontiers in Neurology*, 10, 302. Available at: https://doi.org/10.3389/fneur.2019.00302.

Péloquin, S., Schmierer, K., Leist, T. P., Oh, J., Murray, S. & Lazure, P. (2021) Challenges in multiple sclerosis care: Results from an international mixed-methods study. *Multiple Sclerosis and Related Disorders*, 50, 102854. Available at: https://doi.org/10.1016/j.msard.2021.102854.

Pezzoli, G. & Cereda, E. (2013) Exposure to pesticides or solvents and risk of Parkinson disease. *Neurology*, 80(22), 2035–2041. Available at: https://doi.org/10.1212/WNL.0b013e318294b3c8.

Radder, D., de Vries, N. M., Riksen, N. P., Diamond, S. J., Gross, D., Gold, D. R., Heesakkers, J., Henderson, E., Hommel, A., Lennaerts, H. H., Busch, J., Dorsey, R. E., Andrejack, J. & Bloem, B. R. (2019) Multidisciplinary care for people with Parkinson's disease: The new kids on the block! *Expert Review of Neurotherapeutics*, 19(2), 145–157. Available at: https://doi.org/10.1080/14737175.2019.1561285.

Rajan, R., Brennan, L., Bloem, B. R., Dahodwala, N., Gardner, J., Goldman, J. G., Grimes, D. A., Iansek, R., Kovács, N., McGinley, J., Parashos, S. A., Piemonte, M. & Eggers, C. (2020) Integrated care in Parkinson's disease: A systematic review and meta-analysis. *Movement Disorders*, 35(9), 1509–1531. Available at: https://doi.org/10.1002/mds.28097.

Read, J., Cable, S., Löfqvist, C., Iwarsson, S., Bartl, G. & Schrag, A. (2019) Experiences of health services and unmet care needs of people with late-stage Parkinson's in England: A qualitative study. *PloS One*, 14(12), e0226916. Available at: https://doi.org/10.1371/journal.pone.0226916.

Rietjens, J., Sudore, R. L., Connolly, M., van Delden, J. J., Drickamer, M. A., Droger, M., van der Heide, A., Heyland, D. K., Houttekier, D., Janssen, D., Orsi, L., Payne, S., Seymour, J., Jox, R. J., Korfage, I. J., & European Association for Palliative Care (2017) Definition and recommendations for advance care planning: An international consensus supported by the European Association for Palliative Care. *The Lancet. Oncology*, 18(9), e543–e551. Available at: https://doi.org/10.1016/S1470-2045(17)30582-X.

Ruiz-Lopez, M., Freitas, M. E., Oliveira, L. M., Munhoz, R. P., Fox, S. H., Rohani, M., Rogaeva, E., Lang, A. E. & Fasano, A. (2019) Diagnostic delay in Parkinson's disease caused by PRKN mutations. *Parkinsonism & Related Disorders*, 63, 217–220. Available at: https://doi.org/10.1016/j.parkreldis. 2019.01.010.

Schrag, A., Khan, K., Hotham, S., Merritt, R., Rascol, O. & Graham, L. (2018) Experience of care for Parkinson's disease in European countries: A survey by the European Parkinson's Disease Association. *European Journal of Neurology*, 25, 1410–e120. Available at: https://doi.org/10.1111/ene.13738.

Schwamm, L. H., Chumbler, N., Brown, E., Fonarow, G. C., Berube, D., Nystrom, K., Suter, R., Zavala, M., Polsky, D., Radhakrishnan, K., Lacktman, N., Horton, K., Malcarney, M. B., Halamka, J., Tiner, A. C., & American Heart Association Advocacy Coordinating Committee (2017) Recommendations for the implementation of telehealth in cardiovascular and stroke care: A policy statement from the American Heart Association. *Circulation*, 135(7), e24–e44. Available at: https://doi.org/10.1161/CIR.00000000000 00475.

Shaw, J., Agarwal, P., Desveaux, L., *et al.* (2018) Beyond "implementation": Digital health innovation and service design. *npj Digital Medicine*, 1, 48. Available at: https://doi.org/10.1038/s41746-018-0059-8.

Silva de Lima, A. L., Hahn, T., Evers, L., de Vries, N. M., Cohen, E., Afek, M., Bataille, L., Daeschler, M., Claes, K., Boroojerdi, B., Terricabras, D., Little, M. A., Baldus, H., Bloem, B. R. & Faber, M. J. (2017) Feasibility of large-scale deployment of multiple wearable sensors in Parkinson's disease. *PloS One*, 12(12), e0189161. Available at: https://doi.org/10.1371/journal.pone.0189161.

Soelberg Sorensen, P., Giovannoni, G., Montalban, X., Thalheim, C., Zaratin, P. & Comi, G. (2019) The multiple sclerosis care unit. *Multiple Sclerosis (Houndmills, Basingstoke, England)*, 25(5), 627–636. Available at: https:// doi.org/10.1177/1352458518807082.

Solari, A., Giovannetti, A. M., Giordano, A., Tortorella, C., Torri Clerici, V., Brichetto, G., Granella, F., Lugaresi, A., Patti, F., Salvetti, M., Pesci, I., Pucci, E., Centonze, D., Danni, M. C., Bonavita, S., Ferraro, D., Gallo, A., Gajofatto, A., Nociti, V., Grimaldi, L., ... The ManTra Project (2019) Conversion to secondary progressive multiple sclerosis: Patient awareness and needs. Results from an online survey in Italy and Germany. *Frontiers in Neurology*, 10, 916. Available at: https://doi.org/10.3389/fneur.2019.00916.

Stacey, D., Légaré, F., Col, N. F., Bennett, C. L., Barry, M. J., Eden, K. B., Holmes-Rovner, M., Llewellyn-Thomas, H., Lyddiatt, A., Thomson, R., Trevena, L. & Wu, J. H. (2014) Decision aids for people facing health treatment or screening decisions. *The Cochrane Database of Systematic Reviews*, (1), CD001431. Available at: https://doi.org/10.1002/14651858. CD001431.pub4.

Stroke Alliance for Europe (SAFE) & University of Oxford (2020) At what cost — The economic impact of stroke in Europe. Available at: https://www. safestroke.eu/wp-content/uploads/2020/10/03.-At_What_Cost_EIOS_Full_ Report.pdf.

Suleman, S. & Kim, E. (2015) Decision-making, cognition, and aphasia: Developing a foundation for future discussions and inquiry. *Aphasiology*, 29(12), 1409–1425. Available at: https://doi.org/10.1080/02687038.2015.1049584.

Sylvie, G., Farré Coma, J., Ota, G., Aoife, L., Anna, S., Johanne, S. & Tiago, M. (2021) Co-designing an integrated care network with people living with Parkinson's disease: From patients' narratives to trajectory analysis. *Qualitative Health Research*, 31(14), 2585–2601. Available at: https://doi. org/10.1177/10497323211042605.

Tenison, E., Smink, A., Redwood, S., Darweesh, S., Cottle, H., van Halteren, A., van den Haak, P., Hamlin, R., Ypinga, J., Bloem, B. R., Ben-Shlomo, Y., Munneke, M. & Henderson, E. (2020) Proactive and integrated management and empowerment in Parkinson's disease: Designing a new model of care. *Parkinson's Disease*, 2020, 8673087. Available at: https://doi.org/10.1155/ 2020/8673087.

Trombini, M., Ferraro, F., Iaconi, G., Vestito, L., Bandini, F., Mori, L., Trompetto, C. & Dellepiane, S. (2021) A study protocol for occupational rehabilitation in multiple sclerosis. *Sensors (Basel, Switzerland)*, 21(24), 8436. Available at: https://doi.org/10.3390/s21248436.

UK Government Department of Health (2021) A guide to good practice for digital and data-driven health technologies, updated 19 January 2021. Available at: Available at: https://www.gov.uk/government/publications/code-of-conduct-for-data-driven-health-and-care-technology/initial-code-of-conduct-for-data-driven-health-and-care-technology.

United Nations, Department of Economic and Social Affairs, Population Division (2017) World Population Ageing 2017 — Highlights (ST/ESA/SER.A/397).

van den Heuvel, L., Dorsey, R. R., Prainsack, B., Post, B., Stiggelbout, A. M., Meinders, M. J. & Bloem, B. R. (2020) Quadruple decision making for Parkinson's disease patients: Combining expert opinion, patient preferences, scientific evidence, and big data approaches to reach precision medicine. *Journal of Parkinson's Disease*, 10(1), 223–231. Available at: https://doi. org/10.3233/JPD-191712.

van den Heuvel, L., Meinders, M. J., Post, B., Bloem, B. R. & Stiggelbout, A. M. (2022) Personalizing decision-making for persons with Parkinson's disease: Where do we stand and what to improve? *Journal of Neurology*. Advance online publication. Available at: https://doi.org/10.1007/s00415-022-10969-4.

van der Eijk, M., Faber, M. J., Al Shamma, S., Munneke, M. & Bloem, B. R. (2011) Moving towards patient-centered healthcare for patients with Parkinson's disease. *Parkinsonism & Related Disorders*, 17(5), 360–364. Available at: https://doi.org/10.1016/j.parkreldis.2011.02.012.

van der Eijk, M., Faber, M. J., Ummels, I., Aarts, J. W., Munneke, M. & Bloem, B. R. (2012) Patient-centeredness in PD care: Development and validation of a patient experience questionnaire. *Parkinsonism & Related Disorders*, 18(9), 1011–1016. Available at: https://doi.org/10.1016/j.parkreldis.2012.05.017.

van Halteren, A. D., Munneke, M., Smit, E., Thomas, S., Bloem, B. R. & Darweesh, S. (2020) Personalized care management for persons with Parkinson's disease. *Journal of Parkinson's Disease*, 10(S1), S11–S20. https://doi.org/10.3233/JPD-202126.

van Wamelen, D. J., Sringean, J., Trivedi, D., Carroll, C. B., Schrag, A. E., Odin, P., Antonini, A., Bloem, B. R., Bhidayasiri, R., Chaudhuri, K. R., & International Parkinson and Movement Disorder Society Non Motor Parkinson's Disease Study Group (2021) Digital health technology for non-motor symptoms in people with Parkinson's disease: Futile or future? *Parkinsonism & Related Disorders*, 89, 186–194. Available at: https://doi.org/10.1016/j.parkreldis.2021.07.032.

Venketasubramanian, N., Anderson, C., Ay, H., Aybek, S., Brinjikji, W., de Freitas, G. R., Del Brutto, O. H., Fassbender, K., Fujimura, M., Goldstein, L. B., Haberl, R. L., Hankey, G. J., Heiss, W. D., Lestro Henriques, I., Kase, C. S., Kim, J. S., Koga, M., Kokubo, Y., Kuroda, S., Lee, K., … & Hennerici, M. G. (2021) Stroke care during the COVID-19 pandemic: International expert panel review. *Cerebrovascular Diseases (Basel, Switzerland)*, 50(3), 245–261. Available at: https://doi.org/10.1159/000514155.

Vermersch, P., Faller, A., Czarnota-Szałkowska, D., Meesen, B. & Thalheim, C. (2016) The patient's perspective: How to create awareness for improving access to care and treatment of MS patients? *Multiple Sclerosis (Houndmills, Basingstoke, England)*, 22(2 Suppl), 9–17. Available at: https://doi.org/10.1177/1352458516650742.

Voigt, I., Inojosa, H., Dillenseger, A., Haase, R., Akgün, K. & Ziemssen, T. (2021) Digital twins for multiple sclerosis. *Frontiers in Immunology*, 12, 669811. Available at: https://doi.org/10.3389/fimmu.2021.669811.

Voogdt-Pruis, H. R., Ras, T., van der Dussen, L., *et al.* (2019) Improvement of shared decision making in integrated stroke care: A before and after evaluation using a questionnaire survey. *BMC Health Services Research*, 19, 936. Available at: https://doi.org/10.1186/s12913-019-4761-2.

Wafa, Wolfe, C. D. A., Emmett, E., Roth, G. A., Johnson, C. O. & Wang, Y. (2020) Burden of Stroke in Europe. Thirty-year projections of incidence, prevalence, deaths, and disability-adjusted life years. *Stroke*, 51(8), 2418–2427. Available at: https://doi.org/10.1161/strokeaha.120.029606.

Walton, C., King, R., Rechtman, L., Kaye, W., Leray, E., Marrie, R. A., Robertson, N., La Rocca, N., Uitdehaag, B., van der Mei, I., Wallin, M., Helme, A., Angood Napier, C., Rijke, N. & Baneke, P. (2020) Rising prevalence of multiple sclerosis worldwide: Insights from the Atlas of MS, third edition. *Multiple Sclerosis Journal*, 26(14), 1816–1821. Available at: https://doi.org/10.1177/1352458520970841.

Weisskopf, M. G., Weuve, J., Nie, H., Saint-Hilaire, M. H., Sudarsky, L., Simon, D. K., Hersh, B., Schwartz, J., Wright, R. O. & Hu, H. (2010) Association of cumulative lead exposure with Parkinson's disease. *Environmental Health Perspectives*, 118(11), 1609–1613. Available at: https://doi.org/10.1289/ehp.1002339.

World Health Organization (2020) The top 10 causes of death. WHO's Global Health Estimates Factsheet. Available at: https://www.who.int/news-room/fact-sheets/detail/the-top-10-causes-of-death.

Ypinga, J., Van Halteren, A. D., Henderson, E. J., Bloem, B. R., Smink, A. J., Tenison, E., Munneke, M., Ben-Shlomo, Y. & Darweesh, S. (2021) Rationale and design to evaluate the PRIME Parkinson care model: A prospective observational evaluation of proactive, integrated and patient-centred Parkinson care in The Netherlands (PRIME-NL). *BMC Neurology*, 21(1), 286. Available at: https://doi.org/10.1186/s12883-021-02308-3.

Zhao, J., Li, H., Kung, D., Fisher, M., Shen, Y. & Liu, R. (2020) Impact of the COVID-19 epidemic on stroke care and potential solutions. *Stroke*, 51(7), 1996–2001. Available at: https://doi.org/10.1161/STROKEAHA.120.030225.

Zizzo, N., Bell, E., Lafontaine, A.-L. &s Racine, E. (2017) Examining chronic care patient preferences for involvement in health-care decision making: The case of Parkinson's disease patients in a patient-centred clinic. *Health Expectations*, 20, 655–664. Available at: https://doi.org/10.1111/hex.12497.

Chapter 9

Characterising Redistributed Manufacturing in Healthcare through the Lens of Transdisciplinary Innovation

Dharm Kapletia[*,‡] and Wendy Phillips[†,§]

[*]University of the West of England, Bristol Business School,
Frenchay Campus, Bristol, UK

[†]Trinity College Dublin, Trinity Business School, Dublin, Ireland

[‡]dharm.kapletia@tcd.ie
[§]wendy.phillips@uwe.ac.uk

This chapter explores the emergence of Redistributed Manufacturing (RDM) as a disruptive system that can help address wicked or complex problems in healthcare, which cannot easily be solved by individual disciplines alone. RDM is presented as a new field of practice, whereby a transdisciplinary innovation lens is pivotal for understanding the complexity of the phenomenon and pathways to adoption. This chapter provides the theoretical basis for four critical research propositions to guide future research that robustly considers healthcare system readiness and the evidence base for where to best deploy RDM.

1. Introduction

During much of 2020, critical questions have been raised as to the preparedness of healthcare systems to mount an effective and immediate response to local or national demands and pressures (Capano *et al.*, 2020; O'Flynn, 2020). Healthcare leaders have had to divert resources or transform the delivery of services to ensure they are fit for purpose.

As priorities have changed, much attention has been placed on where to direct investments in innovation and building future resilience into healthcare systems and supply chains (Gereffi, 2020; Woolliscroft, 2020). Historically, the sector was already under long-term pressures to ensure affordable healthcare and deliver solutions to structural issues and increasing instances of complex health conditions (Parekh and Barton, 2010; Sturmberg, Halloran and Martin, 2012). Also, other pressures such as a growing ageing population, cross-border migration and increasing threats of domestic conflict/terrorism have had further impacts on health service priorities and how actors within the healthcare ecosystem can collaborate for best effect.

In this context, healthcare innovations are sought at various levels of analysis — policy, firm (managerial/organisational), service, technological and at the level of end-users and patients (Dopson, Fitzgerald and Ferlie, 2008; Guarcello and de Vargas, 2019). Given the significant systemic nature of the aforementioned challenges, healthcare innovations require a high degree of on-the-ground responsiveness, the ability to ramp up and scale down products and services as needed, the ability to avoid large-scale waste or misdirection of precious resources (medical supplies, staff, infrastructure), and a more targeted approach to meeting the diverse needs of patients (Bigdeli *et al.*, 2013; Remuzat and Toumi, 2016). While considerable attention is rightly placed on the reconfiguration and transformation of front-line services, much of these decisions are dependent on the sourcing and availability of medical supplies and resources. Much of this happens behind the scenes and often only comes to light through media headlines at times of crisis, such as shortages and national/international competition for Personal Protective Equipment (PPE), medical ventilators and medicines (Cohen and van der Meulen Rodgers, 2020; Ortenzi, Albanese and Fadda, 2020). In the context of such complexities, this chapter examines how innovative advances in localised manufacturing can play an instrumental role in transforming future models of healthcare service delivery (Mueller *et al.*, 2020).

An emerging phenomenon known as Redistributed Manufacturing (RDM) has been defined as involving transformation from a 'current state' to a 'future state', typically involving a shift away from large-scale centralised manufacturing towards small-scale decentralised manufacturing and geographically unconstrained supply chains, operating closer to end-users/beneficiaries to produce personalised products on-demand, with less waste and stockpiling (Srai *et al.*, 2016). In healthcare, emerging exemplars include the use of novel production techniques such as additive layer manufacturing, bioprinting, cell microfactories and pharmaceutical factory-in-box, all situated closer to the point of need or use (i.e. in hospitals or regional hubs). Going beyond the focus on a particular technology, for RDM to be implemented, 'system change' is required, with implications across infrastructure, business models, skills, regulations and other key areas (Phillips *et al.*, 2018; Kapletia *et al.*, 2019). The consequences of RDM have the potential to be significant, requiring new concurrent developments across the applied sciences such as business, engineering and medicine to ensure precision quality control across multiple distributed production sites; controlled and auditable touch points between the manufacturing process and the interface with clinicians; and use of new manufacturer service-oriented business models to support working with end-users on product design for the needs of individual patients. This calls for novel conceptual thinking, recognising a multi-faceted form of innovation and going beyond the constraints of academic boundaries and established disciplines.

The concept of transdisciplinarity has been described in part as a response to the increased complexity of contemporary problems in science and technology (Bernstein, 2015). Emerging research in the field of transdisciplinarity has proposed reframing societal needs for solving, mitigating or preventing problems such as violence, disease, environmental pollution and misuse of new technology, whereby new integrated system views and combination of methods provide a richer view of complex problems (Hadorn *et al.*, 2010). This approach is particularly useful for academics, innovators and entrepreneurs contributing to system change (McPhee *et al.*, 2018), providing a greater illumination of the risks and enablers in operational landscape and also hidden connections between different disciplines (Madni, 2007). Interestingly, a transdisciplinary agenda is proposed to support adaptation to *local* conditions in the context of achieving the United Nations Sustainable Development Goals (SDGs) (Moallemi *et al.*, 2020).

In the past two decades, there has been increasing interest in the application of a transdisciplinary lens to the healthcare context, seeking to address complex challenges. For instance, adopting novel mobile health systems (crossing computing, engineering and medical science) (Kumar *et al.*, 2013), and the need for a collaborative research approach to solving the spread of non-communicable diseases (law, public health, health economics and international relations) (Toebes *et al.*, 2020). A transdisciplinary lens can be a powerful tool at any point in the lifecycle of innovation, from early-stage mapping of systemic risk and benefits, to later-stage transformation of operations and support to stakeholders enabling innovation adoption. Bringing together radical advances in manufacturing systems and healthcare delivery, this study contributes to nascent conceptual development of transdisciplinary innovation research (McPhee *et al.*, 2018).

2. Purpose

The purpose of this study is to review how RDM can be considered as a form of transdisciplinary innovation and how insights generated from this analysis can guide (I) future research and (II) practical interventions needed to address complex challenges in healthcare. Literature examining the phenomenon of RDM in healthcare is relatively nascent and few publications have explicitly taken a transdisciplinary innovation lens. Although the focus is on healthcare, this research covers a wider range of literature related to the various dimensions of developing and implementing advanced manufacturing engineering innovations.

For this conceptual chapter, a review of relevant literature and key concepts underpinning RDM and transdisciplinary innovation is conducted. The approach involves identifying key variables from the literature leading towards the development of a conceptual framework, as well as identifying important questions in the field (Wickson, Carew and Russell, 2006). This chapter seeks to advance theory by presenting testable propositions for future RDM in healthcare research and recommendations for further analysis adopting transdisciplinary innovation methods.

3. Redistributed Manufacturing in Healthcare

Existing research in RDM appears to be concentrated in the management and engineering literature bases, where it is explicitly recognised as a phenomenon, yet other terms have been used such as distributed or decentralised manufacturing and reshoring (Srai and Ané, 2016; Harrison, Rafiq and Medcalf, 2018; Theyel, Hofmann and Gregory, 2018). In some studies, at the level of specific technologies such as additive manufacturing, RDM may not be mentioned but is considered in similar fashion as an overarching strategy (Thiesse *et al.*, 2015; Raj *et al.*, 2016; Shukla, Todorov and Kapletia, 2018). Various sectors have been examined such as food production, oil and gas, aerospace, consumer goods and MakerSpace/ MakeSpace workshops (Hennelly *et al.*, 2019; Moreno *et al.*, 2019; Ratnayake, 2019; Veldhuis *et al.*, 2019; Zaki *et al.*, 2019). Within the environmental sustainability literature, RDM is put forward as a manufacturing solution to assist in reducing unnecessary waste and transport as well as associated carbon emissions, and also support the shift towards a circular economy (Freeman, McMahon and Godfrey, 2017; Bessiere, 2019; Godina *et al.*, 2020). The potential impact and functionality of RDM are expected to be augmented when combined with other Industry 4.0 developments, such as intelligent automation and analytics, blockchain and high-speed communications infrastructure.

In the medical/healthcare domain, RDM has been considered as encompassing a range of applications and medical products, including:

- 3D printing (additive manufacturing) of medical devices;
- 3D printing of small molecules (with a single or multiple Active Pharmaceutical Ingredients);
- generating and isolating gasses which act pharmacologically;
- continuous manufacturing (i.e. pharmaceutical factory-in-a-box);
- Advance Therapy Medicinal Product (ATMP) manufacturing and bioprinting (i.e. cell microfactories);
- hybrid manufacturing of combination products (i.e. medical devices with a medicinal component);
- manufacturing of clinical fluids (internal or external use) and blood products.

Over time, these areas of production may be seamlessly combined with other technologies such as diagnostics and biosensing supporting a more integrated time-saving treatment process. Table 1 is not exhaustive, yet it

Table 1.   Emerging RDM literature and transdisciplinary innovation themes.

RDM applications in healthcare	Transdisciplinary innovation themes	Literature
Advanced therapies (cell and gene)	• Decentralised quality control • Regional hub configuration, capabilities and systems integration	Harrison, Rafiq and Medcalf (2018)
Advanced therapies	• Innovator–clinic architecture models — systems analysis of information sharing, chain of custody, co-ownership and reimbursement • Institutional Readiness (IR) — combining systems engineering, business process engineering and biochemical engineering as well as human factors	Medcalf (2021)
Biofabrication (3D and 4D bioprinting and microfluidic devices)	• Materials quality and availability • Biomedical product regulation • Clinical integration of automated platforms	Pavlovich, Hunsberger and Atala (2016)
Biofabrication	• Legal liabilities and regulatory frameworks covering the manufacturing 'process' and final products	Li *et al.* (2020)
Biopharmaceuticals	• Economic viability of targeted biologics produced at required scale and consistency	Evans *et al.* (2021)
Medical devices (personal protective equipment)	• Establishing community-distributed manufacturing and care networks for urgent short-run surge capability, with regulatory oversight and curated design repositories	Manero *et al.* (2020)
Medical devices (wrist splints)	• Clinical and patient involvement in the product design and manufacturing process • Economic modelling of transformed clinical practices using 3D printer technologies and international comparisons	Paterson *et al.* (2015)
Pharmaceuticals (small molecules)	• Value chain reconfiguration using advanced manufacturing and continuous manufacturing technologies	Harrington, Phillips and Srai (2017)
Pharmaceuticals (small molecules, portable drug synthesiser)	• Quality assurance for switching between products and dosage, using both automated and human controls • Advances in downstream processing and dispensing, configured to meet clinical requirements and discovery	Adamo *et al.* (2016)

illustrates the diversity of themes related to transdisciplinary innovation, which require further research to support RDM translation into practice as well as realisation of clinical benefit.

4. Theoretical Foundation and Hypothesis Development

Redistributed Manufacturing in healthcare can be presented as a new transdisciplinary field of practice, whereby new knowledge is formed via the integration of specialist domains (as illustrated in Figure 1), including (but not limited to) Policy and Regulation, Medical Science, Precision Manufacturing Engineering, Business and Management and Digital Design or Computer Aided Design (CAD) (McPhee *et al.*, 2018; Phillips *et al.*, 2018; Rantanen and Khinast, 2015). We propose that RDM in healthcare has a significant role to play in the future in solving the pressing challenge of ensuring a resilient and environmentally sustainable supply of medical products, and will also be instrumental in enabling the delivery of personalised medicine. Furthermore, the two-way arrow in Figure 1 indicates the dynamic learning and adaptation loop between innovators involved in either the development or output/impact of RDM, which lends itself to ongoing product-based services.

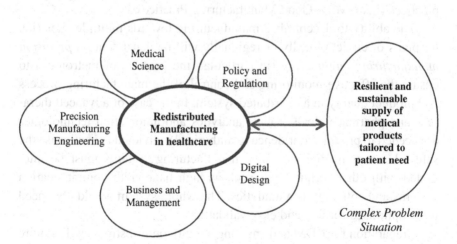

Figure 1.   Conceptualising Redistributed Manufacturing in healthcare (modified from McPhee, Bliemel and Bijl-Brouwer, 2018).

Taking a high-level *policy and regulatory* view, the extent to which governance frameworks in healthcare keep pace with innovative technological developments related to RDM will affect potential translation into practice and future market potential for industrial innovators. The UK Medicines and Healthcare products Regulatory Agency (MHRA) has been actively engaged in developing a new regulatory framework for point-of-care manufacturing, i.e. the production of healthcare products and therapies close to where they are needed and similarly the European regulator (EMA) cites the need to adapt future regulatory science to consider such advances in manufacturing technologies: all of which will provide much-needed guidance for innovators working across technical and managerial domains (EMA, 2018; MHRA, 2018).

Breakthroughs in the *medical sciences* are providing new opportunities, such as the ability to treat complex conditions with advanced therapeutics using living cells to restore normal body function and the combination of leading-edge real-time diagnostics and bio-sensing with local production for a faster solution (i.e. 3D printed orthosis, prothesis) (Whyte and Gillespie, 2019; Medcalf, 2021). Such developments have significant implications for healthcare infrastructure and management, which will need to allow for design, processing manufacturing and support facilities near to patients which adhere to strict quality standards and practices (i.e. GMP – Good Manufacturing Practice).

The ability to decentralise manufacturing towards multiple sites (i.e. hospitals or clinics) locally or regionally will be dependent on *precision manufacturing engineering* (in particular, the practice of metrology) to ensure the effective monitoring and control of the manufacturing process and product quality in a distributed system. In the case of advanced therapies and pharmaceuticals, robust analytics and automation technologies are needed to provide confidence to authorised individuals to authorise the safe release of medicines. Thus, manufacturing systems must be integrated with other technologies such as high bandwidth communication systems and software data analytics. The whole system would also need to be optimised for fast and easy validation.

Preparation for RDM and ensuring a return on investment will require effective *business* practices and *management* of associated transformation programmes and projects, within the healthcare system. This will require mapping the new configuration of industrial and clinical roles, responsibilities and processes, particularly the chain of custody for medicinal products, as well as how new risks and dependencies will be managed (Medcalf, 2021; Stindt *et al.*, 2016). Managerial expertise will also be required to consider alternative reimbursement models and consider value, pricing and costing of the whole redistributed system — requiring greater transparency between manufacturer and service provider (Banda, Tait and Mittra, 2018).

In an overlap with the medical sciences and precision manufacturing engineering, *digital design* has a crucial role to play at various levels of analysis. In particular, digital manufacturing innovation creates the opportunity to model and simulate a redistributed manufacturing system within a healthcare context before it goes into operation. Once installed, manufacturing designers and clinicians can work collaboratively to co-design product solutions or optimise the production process to meet demand. The advantage of manufacturing at the point of care is the proximity to patients, which allows for greater feedback and design customisation to suit individual needs.

4.1. *Advancing the research agenda*

Existing research in RDM primarily concentrates on advancing a specific discipline, with the aim of building on past theory and providing case exemplars of how new advanced manufacturing technologies would transform existing operations in practice (Phillips *et al.*, 2018; Srai *et al.*, 2016, 2020). Many of these studies have also focused on documenting early-stage findings, setting out calls for further research and investment. Similarly, research and innovation funding seeks to advance technical understanding and knowledge within the narrow frame of a particular discipline, such as additive manufacturing and advanced therapies (Engineering), or supply chain and logistics (Business and Management).

RDM, however, offers a rich context for future empirical studies that adopt a transdisciplinary innovation lens. Solving a complex problem situation through transdisciplinary innovation such as the emergency supply of medical products (as stated in Figure 1) will result in new knowledge through the integration of individual disciplines and is expected to contribute learning back to those disciplines (McPhee, Bliemel and Bijl-Brouwer, 2018). Furthermore, there is a need to better understand how the inherent unpredictability of transdisciplinary working is coordinated to achieve innovation. Given the systemic nature of transdisciplinary innovation, it is also necessary to consider how impact is measured and what this offers above and beyond traditional methods and measures, such as shifting from efficacy to long-term recovery (Archibald *et al.*, 2018).

Given the early stage of maturity for most RDM in healthcare innovations and the need for further research and analysis at the intersection of the disciplines cited in Figure 1, we argue that the following propositions should be explored.

Proposition **1 — Platforms and infrastructure required for RDM are radically different from centralised manufacturing.** To justify the investment in RDM, manufacturing technologies must clearly demonstrate value for money and offer patient benefit that is likely to coalesce around the promise of on-demand personalised medicine. This has implications for the clarity and creativity of new value propositions underpinning RDM. From a transdisciplinary innovation perspective, this requires RDM production platforms to deliver at pace and flexibly to meet a variety of patient needs/requirements rather than relying on bulk procurement and stored inventory from mass production. It also requires a number of major infrastructure considerations, such as financial investment in new production facilities, high-skills design, automation and manufacturing training, and cross-disciplinary collaboration to establish new processes that satisfy quality standards (ISO, GMP, etc.). With a shift from the specialisation associated with centralised production to a transdisciplinary RDM environment, we expect staff operating at the point of care to have stronger expertise in systems engineering and the practice of (multi-organisational) systems integration between manufacturing and medicine. We posit that for the most part, the development of such expertise constitutes a novel development, which may lead to new opportunities to improve overall quality of healthcare provisioning.

Proposition **2 — Assurance of quality and safety for the production of medical products in an RDM system requires new capabilities**

for operators of production platforms. Linking production platforms to the demands of healthcare operating environments, there is a critical need to ensure product reproducibility, comparability and compliance. This has implications, on the one hand, for manufacturers of production platforms to better support post-production verification, and, on the other hand, for operators (where manufacturers are not involved) who will need to work with novel and rapid quantitative analytical methodologies and characterisation technologies. These considerations require close ongoing collaboration between experts, particularly where novel products are produced in response to needs arising from personalised medicine. For technology developers, the need to support interoperability between emerging hardware and software technologies (including between diagnosis and production) will also require diverse collaboration between engineers, scientists, designers and clinical analysts.

Proposition 3 — **Manufacturing at the point of care presents a major challenge to existing regulatory and governance frameworks and is a barrier to innovation adoption.** The issues raised by Proposition 2 concerning the assurance of quality and safety in combination with the need to have an effective audit process raise important questions about the optimal product approval pathway, as well as legal and regulatory responsibilities in any shared chain of custody. Conventional quality systems and regulatory paradigms based on centralised production and testing are not easily adapted for use in RDM environments. Also, it is not practical for each hospital, clinic or other sites in a distributed production system to hold separate manufacturing authorisations. Operating across geographical jurisdictions and ensuring suitable staff with quality and regulatory expertise are available across dispersed sites also present further challenges for point-of-care manufacturing.

Proposition 4 — **RDM requires innovative transdisciplinary frameworks to support the justification and evidence base for healthcare service transformation and realisation of new business models.** A simple comparison of procuring medical products using existing methods vs RDM technologies is misleading and would lack an appreciation of the practical complexities involved. A more sophisticated systems-level analysis is required and novel transdisciplinary frameworks are needed to cognitively recognise and communicate across disciplines affected by any shift towards RDM, including (but not limited to):

- redesigned healthcare service architectures (i.e. business process models and touch points between products and services, supply chain and inventory flows) centered around point-of-care manufacturing and patient need;
- life cycle analysis of RDM-based medical products covering material inputs, logistics, production, post-production finishing, clinical use and disposal or re-use/re-engineering/recycling;
- analysis of whole system RDM product costs, which factors in the variability associated with personalised medicine and clinical dependencies (i.e. intangible hidden costs, particularly staff inputs);
- audit of new staff and skills/training, and new equipment and infrastructure, across organisational boundaries;
- novel commercial agreements based on closer relationships between manufacturer and healthcare service provider, likely to include incentives/rewards for achieving patient benefits and apportioning system-level risk and cost controls/reduction.

The practical representation of such analyses may also benefit from applying novel methodologies such as simulation studies to improve understanding across disciplines, both pre- and post-adoption (Davis, Eisenhardt and Bingham, 2007). Moving towards conducting more quantitative analyses, we expect a transdisciplinary innovation lens to yield greater insights when testing hypotheses related to whether RDM:

- improves the availability of medical products in both (I) business as usual and (II) emergency scenarios;
- results in improved patient outcomes over varied timeframes;
- leads to lower environmental impact (i.e. lower pollution or carbon emissions) and a move towards more sustainable approaches to healthcare manufacturing;
- reduces waste in terms of patient and clinical time, as well as systemic resources needed to produce physical products.

Looking across these areas, a critical analysis is also needed to assess where RDM does not offer any clear immediate benefits or the timing is not yet right (i.e. maturity of system technologies and dependencies, etc.). Such insights can help prioritise healthcare investment and resources according to where it is most likely to yield benefit.

5. Discussion

Using the lens of transdisciplinary innovation, we observe RDM as an emerging new field of practice. Building on scant research, which has predominately focused on the 'potential' of RDM, this chapter calls for further research to more robustly examine cross-disciplinary prepared-ness of the healthcare system and where to best deploy RDM for the greatest effect. Future research in this area requires close collaboration between scholars and healthcare professionals working towards a shared understanding of how new models of delivery will be realised in practice.

Transdisciplinary innovation provides a novel analytical approach, particularly where an integrated system perspective is required to help understand factors affecting innovation development, adoption and per-formance in use. Advances in transdisciplinary innovation methodolo-gies have the potential to generate powerful insights in complex settings such as healthcare provision and help guide the introduction of new systems and technologies such as RDM. We call for further studies to apply models and frameworks from the innovation literature to advance our understanding of RDM. For instance, technology roadmapping meth-odologies may provide the ability to map connections across disciplines with a view to deliberatively identifying and co-creating new areas for collaboration and (cross-boundary) partnering that are essential for innovation.

We expect transdisciplinary innovation to offer further impactful insights related to other chapters covered in this book, particularly in the context of introducing new healthcare technologies and building innova-tion capability within healthcare services.

5.1. *Future models*

Where adopted, RDM has the potential to bridge the feedback loop (in close to real time) between R&D — production — clinical application — patient impact, which fixes a fundamental weakness with the current disjointed system across a range of medical products and therapies (i.e. manufacturers not having visibility of the efficacy or consequences of their products in use) (Andrews *et al.*, 2020; Medcalf, 2021; Nicolini *et al.*, 2008; Yip, Phaal and Probert, 2015). The importance of this cannot be understated as a potential transformational shift in how healthcare is delivered and improved. Furthermore, with this in mind, in cases where RDM is fully adopted, this will also result in structural changes to existing industrial supply relationships. Disintermediation of existing healthcare supply chains by new entrants may be possible, seizing channel control of healthcare providers and providing new value propositions to Payors or Commissioners and healthcare procurement bodies. Establishing optimal future configuration models requires transdisciplinary collaboration which crosses the divides of medicine, engineering and business.

Recent research tells us that manufacturer incumbents may need to adopt dual business models to survive new competition from dedicated RDM providers (Christensen, Waldeck and Fogg, 2017; Roscoe and Blome, 2019). The restructuring of such relationships may well depend on the (post-COVID-19) leadership and attitude to innovation (i.e. risk appetite) of healthcare service providers as well as the buyers and end-users of medical products (Heinonen and Strandvik, 2020). We argue against a return to previous models of risk management. Where RDM is considered as part of future risk mitigation strategy, there is an opportunity to build greater resilience into healthcare systems — thus a range of stakeholder views must be incorporated into the business case of RDM.

We also expect that by taking a transdisciplinary innovation lens, future research is expected to generate insights back to specialist disciplines, such as health economics and systems engineering. For applications where RDM presents a serious proposition, we expect future analyses to consider the costs and benefits of a suite of medical products that can be produced on the same platform(s), as well as sharing among multiple hospital/clinic sites as a regional local manufacturing capability.

Acknowledgements

This research was funded by the Redistributed Manufacturing in Healthcare Network (RiHN). The RiHN was awarded a $2m grant from the UK Engineering and Physical Sciences Research Council (EPSRC) (Ref. EP/T014970/1), which commenced in July 2020.

References

Adamo, A., Beingessner, R. L., Behnam, M., Chen, J., Jamison, T. F., Jensen, K. F., Monbaliu, J. C. M., Myerson, A. S., Revalor, E. M., Snead, D. R. & Stelzer, T. (2016) On-demand continuous-flow production of pharmaceuticals in a compact, reconfigurable system. *Science*, 352(6281), 61–67.

Andrews, R., Greasley, D., Knight, S., Sireau, S., Jordan, A., Bell, A. & White, P. (2020) Collaboration for clinical innovation: A nursing and engineering alliance for better patient care. *Journal of Research in Nursing*, 25(3), 291–304.

Archibald, M. M., Lawless, M., Lawless, M., Harvey, G. & Kitson, A. L. (2018) Transdisciplinary research for impact: Protocol for a realist evaluation of the relationship between transdisciplinary research collaboration and knowledge translation. *BMJ Open*, 8(4), e021775.

Banda, G., Tait, J. & Mittra, J. (2018) Evolution of business models in regenerative medicine: Effects of a disruptive innovation on the innovation ecosystem. *Clinical Therapeutics*, 40(7), 1084–1094.

Bernstein, J. (2015) Transdisciplinarity: A review of its origins, development, and current issues. *Journal of Research Practice*, 11(1), 1–20.

Bessiere, D., Charnley, F., Tiwari, A. & Moreno, M. A. (2019) A vision of redistributed manufacturing for the UK's consumer goods industry. *Production Planning & Control*, 30(7), 555–567.

Bigdeli, M., Jacobs, B., Tomson, G., Laing, R., Ghaffar, A., Dujardin, B. & Van Damme, W. (2013) Access to medicines from a health system perspective. *Health Policy and Planning*, 28(7), 692–704.

Capano, G., Howlett, M., Darryl, S. L., Jarvis, M., Goyal, R. & Goyal, N. (2020) Mobilizing policy (in)capacity to fight COVID-19: Understanding variations in state responses. *Policy and Society*, 39(3), 285–308.

Christensen, C., Waldeck, A. & Fogg, R. (2017) How disruptive innovation can finally revolutionize healthcare. *Industry Horizons*: *Innosight Executive Briefings*, Spring.

Cohen, J. & van der Meulen Rodgers, Y. (2020) Contributing factors to personal protective equipment shortages during the COVID-19 pandemic. *Preventative Medicine*, 141, 106263.

Davis, J. P., Eisenhardt, K. M. & Bingham, C. B. (2007) Developing theory through simulation methods. *Academy of Management Review*, 32(2), 480–499.

Dopson, S., Fitzgerald, L. & Ferlie, E. (2008) Understanding change and innovation in healthcare settings: Reconceptualizing the active role of context. *Journal of Change Management*, 8(3–4), 213–231.

EMA (2018) EMA Regulatory Science to 2025: Reference Material, Scientific Committees Regulatory Science Strategy, European Medicines Agency. Published 23 October 2018.

Evans, S. E., Harrington, T., Rodriguez Rivero, M. C., Rognin, E., Tuladhar, T. & Daly, R. (2021) 2D and 3D inkjet printing of biopharmaceuticals — A review of trends and future perspectives in research and manufacturing. *International Journal of Pharmaceutics*, 599.

Freeman, R., McMahon, C. & Godfrey, P. (2017) An exploration of the potential for re-distributed manufacturing to contribute to a sustainable, resilient city. *International Journal of Sustainable Engineering*, 10(4–5), 260–271.

Gereffi, G. (2020) What does the COVID-19 pandemic teach us about global value chains? The case of medical supplies. *Journal of International Business Policy*, 3, 287–301.

Godina, R., Ribeiro, I., Matos, F., Ferreira, B. T., Carvalho, H. & Peças, P. (2020) Impact assessment of additive manufacturing on sustainable business models in Industry 4.0 context. *Sustainability*, 12(17), 7066.

Guarcello, C. & de Vargas, E. R. (2020) Service innovation in healthcare: A systematic literature review. *Latin American Business Review*, 21(4), 353–369.

Hadorn, G. H., Pohl, C. & Bammer, G. (2010) *Solving Problems through Transdisciplinary Research*. The Oxford Handbook of Interdisciplinarity. pp. 431–452.

Harrington, T., Phillips, M. A. & Srai, J. (2017) Reconfiguring global pharmaceutical value networks through targeted technology interventions. *International Journal of Production Research*, 55(5), 1471–1487.

Harrison, R. P., Rafiq, Q. A. & Medcalf, N. (2018) Centralised versus decentralised manufacturing and the delivery of healthcare products: A United Kingdom exemplar. *Cytotherapy*, 20(6), 873–890.

Heinonen, K. & Strandvik, T. (2020) Reframing service innovation: COVID-19 as a catalyst for imposed service innovation. *Journal of Service Management*, 32(1), 101–112.

Hennelly, P. A., Srai, J. S., Graham, G., Meriton, R. & Kumar, M. (2017) Do makerspaces represent scalable production models of community-based redistributed manufacturing? *Production Planning & Control*, 30(7), 540–554.

Kapletia, D., Phillips, W., Medcalf, D., Makatsoris, H., McMahon, C. & Rich, N. (2019) Redistributed manufacturing — Challenges for operations management. *Production Planning & Control*, 30(7), 493–495.

Kumar, S., Nilsen, W. J., Abernethy, A., Atienza, A., Patrick, K., Pavel, M., Riley, W. T., Shar, A., Spring, B., Spruijt-Metz, D., Hedeker, D., Honavar, V., Kravitz, R., Craig, R., Lefebvre, C., Mohr, D. C., Murphy, S. A., Quinn, C., Shusterman, V. & Swendeman, D. (2013) Mobile health technology evaluation: The mHealth evidence workshop. *American Journal of Preventative Medicine*, 45(2), 228–236.

Li, P., Faulkner, A. & Medcalf, N. (2020) 3D bioprinting in a 2D regulatory landscape: Gaps, uncertainties, and problems. *Law, Innovation and Technology*, 12(1), 1–29.

Manero, A., Smith, P., Koontz, A., Dombrowski, M., Sparkman, J., Courbin, D. & Chi, A. (2020) Leveraging 3D printing capacity in times of crisis: Recommendations for COVID-19 distributed manufacturing for medical equipment rapid response. *International Journal of Environmental Research and Public Health*, 17, 4634.

McPhee, C., Bliemel, M. & van der Bijl-Brouwer, M. (2018) Editorial: Transdisciplinary innovation. *Technology Innovation Management Review*, 8(8), 3–6.

Medcalf, N. (2021) Re-engineering the innovator–clinic interface for adoption of advanced therapies. *Future Medicine*, 16(3), 295–308.

MHRA (2018) Life Sciences Industrial Strategy Update, The Medicines and Healthcare Products Regulatory Agency, UK Government.

Moallemi, E. A., Malekpour, S., Hadjikakou, M., Raven, R., Szetey, K., Ningrum, D., Dhiaulhaq, A. & Bryan, B. A. (2020) Achieving the sustainable development goals requires transdisciplinary innovation at the local scale. *One Earth*, 3(3), 300–313.

Moreno, M., Court, R., Wright, M. & Charnley, F. (2019) Opportunities for redistributed manufacturing and digital intelligence as enablers of a circular economy. *International Journal of Sustainable Engineering*, 12(2), 77–94.

Mueller, T., Elkaseer, A., Charles, A., Fauth, J., Rabsch, D., Scholz, A., Marquardt, C., Nau, K. & Scholz, S. G. (2020) Eight weeks later — The unprecedented rise of 3D printing during the COVID-19 pandemic — A case study, lessons learned, and implications on the future of global decentralized manufacturing. *Applied Sciences*, 10(12), 4135.

Nicolini, D., Powell, J., Conville, P. & Martinez-Solano, L. (2008) Managing knowledge in the healthcare sector: A review. *International Journal of Management Reviews*, 10(3), 245–263.

O'Flynn, J. (2020) Confronting the big challenges of our time: Making a difference during and after COVID-19. *Public Management Review*, 23(7), 961–980.

Ortenzi, F., Albanese, E. & Fadda, M. (2020) A transdisciplinary analysis of COVID-19 in Italy: The most affected country in Europe. *International Journal of Environmental Research and Public Health*, 17(24), 9488.

Parekh, A. K. & Barton, M. B. (2010) The challenge of multiple comorbidity for the US health care system. *JAMA*, 303(13), 1303–1304.

Paterson, A. M., Bibb, R., Campbell, I. & Bingham, G. (2015) Comparing additive manufacturing technologies for customised wrist splints. *Rapid Prototyping Journal*, 21(3), 230–243.

Pavlovich, M. J., Hunsberger, J. & Atala, A. (2016) Biofabrication: A secret weapon to advance manufacturing, economies, and healthcare. *Trends in Biotechnology*, 34(9), 679–680.

Phillips, W., Medcalf, N., Dalgarno, K., Makatoris, H., Sharples, S., Srai, J., Hourd, P. & Kapletia, D. (2018) Redistributed manufacturing in healthcare: Creating new value through disruptive innovation. EPSRC Redistributed Manufacturing in Healthcare Network.

Raj, B., Gregory, M. & Tiwari, M. K. (2016) Editorial note on the special issue of "Distributed Manufacturing to Enhance Productivity". *International Journal of Production Research*, 54(23), 6913–6916.

Rantanen, J. & Khinast, J. (2015) The future of pharmaceutical manufacturing sciences. *Journal of Pharmaceutical Sciences*, 104(11), 3612–3638.

Ratnayake, C. (2019) Enabling RDM in challenging environments via additive layer manufacturing: Enhancing offshore petroleum asset operations. *Production Planning & Control*, 30(7), 522–539.

Remuzat, C. & Toumi, M. (2016) PHP323 — Health care system inefficiencies related to medicines: Any potential room for improvement? *Value in Health*, 19(7), A497.

Roscoe, S. & Blome, C. (2019) Understanding the emergence of redistributed manufacturing: An ambidexterity perspective. *Production Planning & Control*, 30(7), 496–509.

Shukla, M., Todorov, I. & Kapletia, D. (2018) Application of additive manufacturing for mass customisation: Understanding the interaction of critical barriers. *Production Planning & Control*, 29(10), 814–825.

Srai, J. S. & Ane, C. (2015) Institutional and strategic operations perspectives on manufacturing reshoring. *International Journal of Production Research*, 54(23), 7193–7211.

Srai, J. S., Kumar, M., Graham, G., Phillips, W., Tooze, J., Ford, S., Beecher, P., Raj, B., Gregory, M., Tiwari, M. K., Ravi, B., Neely, A., Shankar, R., Charnley, F. & Tiwari, A. (2016) Distributed manufacturing: Scope, challenges and opportunities. *International Journal of Production Research*, 54(23), 6917–6935.

Stindt, D., Sahamie, R., Nuss, C. & Tuma, A. (2016) How transdisciplinarity can help to improve operations research on sustainable supply chains — A transdisciplinary modeling framework. *Journal of Business Logistics*, 37(2), 113–131.

Sturmberg, J. P., O'Halloran, D. M. & Martin, C. M. (2012) Healthcare reform: The need for a complex adaptive systems approach. In: Sturmberg, J. P. & Martin, C. M. (eds.) *Handbook of Systems and Complexity in Health*. Springer, New York, pp. 827–853.

Theyel, G., Hofmann, K. & Gregory, M. (2018) Understanding manufacturing location decision making: Rationales for retaining, offshoring, reshoring, and hybrid approaches. *Economic Development Quarterly*, 32(4), 300–312.

Thiesse, F., Wirth, M., Kemper, H. G., Moisa, M., Morar, D., Heiner, L., Piller, F., Buxmann, P., Mortara, L., Ford, S. & Minshall, T. (2015) Economic implications of additive manufacturing and the contribution of MIS. *Business Information Systems Engineering*, 57(2), 139–148.

Toebes, B., Hesselman, M., Mierau, J. O. & van Dijk, J. P. (2020) A renewed call for transdisciplinary action on NCDs. *BMC International Health and Human Rights*, 20(22), 22.

Veldhuis, A. J., Glover, J., Bradley, D., Behzadian, K., López-Avilés, A., Cottee, J., Downing, C., Ingram, J., Leach, M., Farmani, R., Butler, D., Pike, A., De Propris, L., Purvis, L., Robinson, P. & Yang, A. (2019) Re-distributed manufacturing and the food-water-energy nexus: Opportunities and challenges. *Production Planning and Control*, 30(7), 593–609.

Whyte, J. & Gillespie, J. (2019) How precision medicine impacts patient-centricity in clinical trials. *Clinical Leader*. Guest Column, published 5 July 2019.

Wickson, F., Carew, A. L. & Russell, A. W. (2006) Transdisciplinary research: Characteristics, quandaries and quality. *Futures*, 38(9), 1046–1059.

Woolliscroft, J. O. (2020) Innovation in response to the COVID-19 pandemic crisis. *Academic Medicine, Journal of the Association of American Medical Colleges*, 95(8), 1140–1142.

Yip, M. H., Phaal, R. & Probert, D. (2015) Stakeholder engagement in early stage product-service system development for healthcare informatics. *Engineering Management Journal*, 26(3), 52–62.

Zaki, M., Theodoulidis, B., Shapira, P., Neely, A. & Friedrich, M. T. (2019) Redistributed manufacturing and the impact of Big Data: A consumer goods perspective. *Production Planning & Control*, 30(7), 568–581.

Index

Series on Technology Management

(Continuation of series card page)